BUILDING THE CLASSIC PHYSIQUE THE NATURAL WAY

By
STEVE REEVES
with
John Little,
George Helmer and
Bob Wolff, Ph.D.

Precautionary Advice

This book is intended for informational and educational purposes only. Individuals should always consult their physician before beginning or altering an exercise program. Resistance exercises can be done safely if proper form and appropriate weights are used; readers must use common sense to make sure both conditions are met at all times.

2nd Edition

Copyright® 1996 by Steve Reeves International Inc.

All rights reserved including the right of reproduction in whole or in part in any form.

Published by: Steve Reeves International Inc.
PO Bos 3547, Mission Viejo, CA 92690

Printed by: Abbey Graphics
1631 Clark Street, Unit 102
Arcadia, California 91006

Text layout and design:
Jackie Frahm, Abbey Graphics

Cover design: George Helmer

Copy editor: Terri Daxon, Daxon Writing Service

Photos courtesy of David Chapman Archives, Milton T. Moore Jr. Archives and the Steve Reeves Archives.

Manufactured in the United States of America

Library of Congress Cataloguing Information:
Reeves, Steve
BUILDING THE CLASSIC PHYSIQUE
The Natural Way
1. Fitness/health I. Title
Soft Cover: ISBN: 1-885096-10-0
Hard Cover: ISBN: 1-885096-11-9

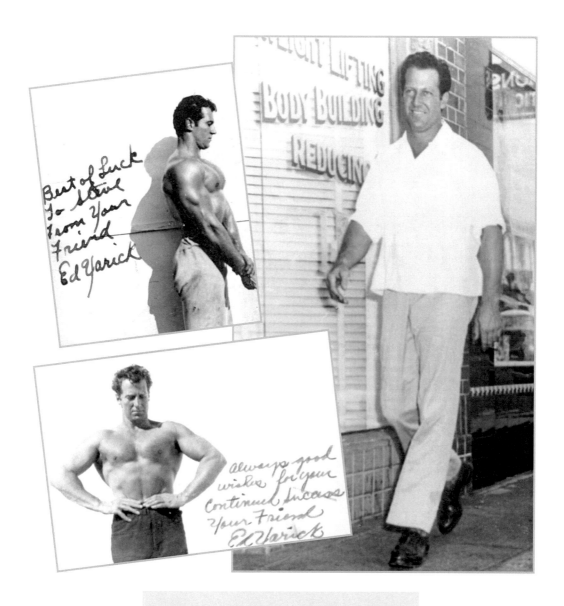

DEDICATION

I would like to dedicate this book to my mentor, Ed Yarick. Ed was a very imposing man, standing 6-foot-4-inches and weighing in at a rock-solid 240 pounds. With his perpetual bronze tan, blond hair and blue eyes, he looked like a Viking prince. Yarick was an outstanding male role model for a teenage boy. He was a giving person with great integrity and had a terrific sense of humor. Yarick was too young to be my father and too old to be my brother, but he did a real good job at doubling as both. Ed was the nicest guy I have ever known and the best friend I ever had.

Acknowledgments and Thanks

With special thanks––

To George Helmer for his extraordinary research and help with the 1st and 2nd editions. To photographers Tony Lanza, Russ Warner and Paul Stone Raymor who took the majority of the bodybuilding photographs featured in this book.

To David Chapman and Milton T. Moore Jr. for providing photograph copies from their collections.

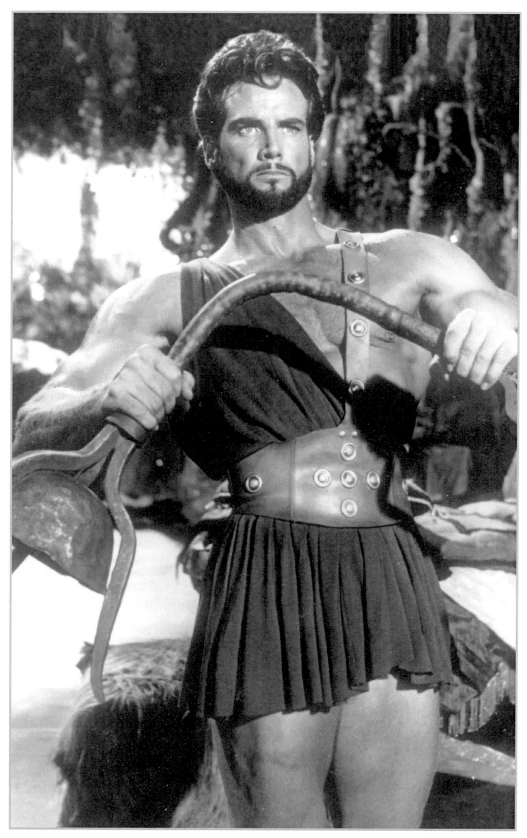

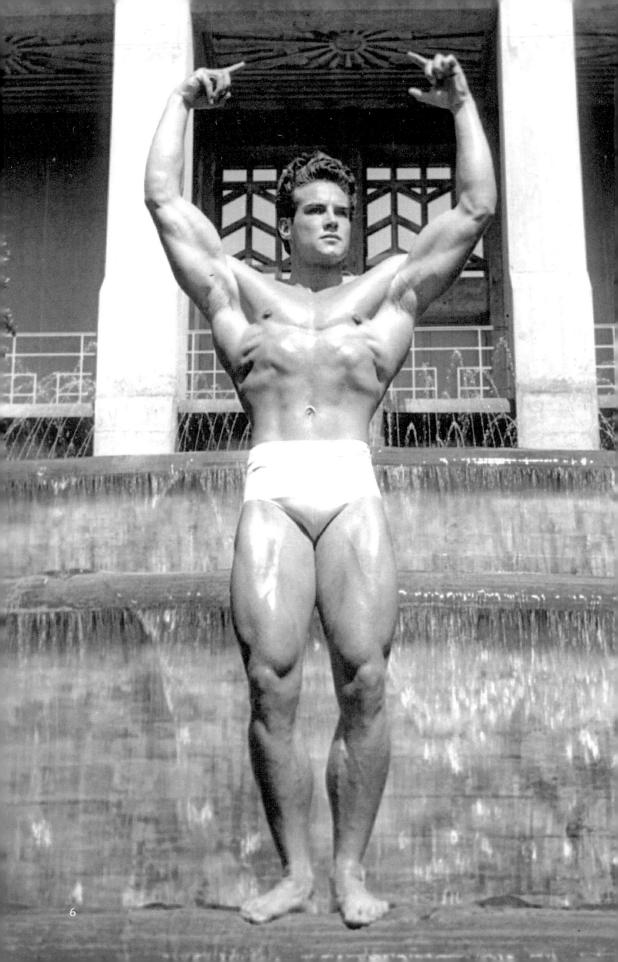

Contents

INTRODUCTION by John Little
PREFACE by Bob Wolff, Ph.D.
FOREWORD by Armand Tanny

PART ONE:
MY LIFE IN BODYBUILDING

- 14 Chapter 1: On the Shoulders of Giants
- 17 Chapter 2: Moving Forward
- 19 Chapter 3: Go West, Young Man
- 21 Chapter 4: I Discover Bodybuilding
- 24 Chapter 5: Enter Ed Yarick
- 30 Chapter 6: Life in the Service
- 34 Chapter 7: My Bodybuilding Career Begins!

PART TWO:
THE SCIENCE OF BODYBUILDING

- 46 Chapter 8: Preliminary Considerations
- 51 Chapter 9: No Brain, No Gain
- 55 Chapter 10: Training Logic
- 59 Chapter 11: High-Intensity Training
- 63 Chapter 12: Building the Classic Physique — First Principles
- 66 Chapter 13: What Is the "Classic Physique"?
- 73 Chapter 14: Building the Classic Physique — the Routine
- 88 Chapter 15: Training the Midsection
- 90 Chapter 16: Maximum Muscular Development

PART THREE:
ADDITIONAL TRAINING CONSIDERATIONS

- 94 Chapter 17: Super High-Intensity Training
- 97 Chapter 18: The Pyramid System
- 98 Chapter 19: Exercising in Opposition
- 103 Chapter 20: Circuit Training for the Executive
- 105 Chapter 21: A Training Program for Seniors
- 107 Chapter 22: Muscle Control — and the Art of Posing
- 115 Chapter 23: The Power of Walking
- 127 Chapter 24: Getting Smart about Nutrition
- 135 Chapter 25: Losing Body Fat
- 139 Chapter 26: Rules to Live By

PART FOUR:
QUESTIONS AND ANSWERS

- 142 Chapter 27: A Bodybuilding Seminar with Steve Reeves

APPENDIXES

- 177 1. My Handwritten Championship Workout
- 181 2. My Favorite Bodybuilding Exercises
- 201 3. Steve Reeves' Bodybuilding Principles
- 203 4. Awards and Honors Bestowed Upon Steve Reeves
- 207 5. The Search for Bodybuilding's "Holy Grail" — Steve Reeves' Garage Workout by George Helmer
- 211 6. What the Press Said about Steve Reeves
- 231 7. In their own Words — Impressions of Steve Reeves from Mentors and Friends

Introduction

"A few days before the contest we heard rumors about a man that had throngs of people following him along the Lake Michigan beach front, and we could not imagine who could draw crowds by merely walking along a beach."

— George Eiferman, 1947 (referring to Steve Reeves)

The book you are now holding in your hands represents the distilled wisdom of the greatest bodybuilder the world has ever seen. Without question, the knowledge contained within its pages will put you well on your way to developing what Steve Reeves terms, "The Classic Physique."

I first met Steve back in 1986 — when he was 60 years of age — and his physical condition blew me away. I'd seen most of his films on television and been similarly impressed with both his physique and how he carried himself.

Some have called him "A man's man," and this is probably true — for Steve Reeves has lived life on his own terms, without compromising one single value, since day one. At the height of his movie career, he turned his back on Hollywood to build a ranch and raise Morgan horses (a lifelong passion). He lives primarily on the food he grows on his own property and continues his bodybuilding training with a passion and a strength that has left many of those half his age gasping to keep pace.

I've met and interviewed virtually every top bodybuilding champion of the past two decades — from Dorian Yates to Arnold Schwarzenegger — and not one of them has made the impact upon me that Steve Reeves has. The man is a walking encyclopedia of bodybuilding wisdom and now — finally! — he's decided to let us in on what natural bodybuilding is really all about.

Reeves competed in a day when steroids and other muscle growth-stimulating drugs were unheard of, which means that the incredible body you see gracing the pages of this publication is all natural and serves as a beacon of what is possible for human beings if they're willing to put forth the dedication and commitment to pursuing physical excellence.

More and more people who are involved in bodybuilding, from the first-time amateur to the seasoned professional, are looking to the physique of a man born in Glasgow, Montana on January 21, 1926 as the standard by which to measure physical perfection. That the Reeves' physique has influenced thousands of bodybuilders the world over is a fact. That it continues to do so, particularly in light of the quality of competitive physiques today, is nothing short of astounding! Nevertheless, this is indeed the case.

In his inspirational book, *Steve Reeves: One of a Kind*, Milton Moore Jr. has collected hundreds of testimonials from professional athletes such as Jesse Owens, Willie Mays, Harmon Killebrew and Rocky Bleier. Hollywood has paid homage with glowing tributes from luminaries such as Bob Hope, James Cagney, Bo Derek, Clint Walker, Burt Reynolds, Sylvestor Stallone, Arnold Schwarzenegger and Lou Ferrigno — to name but a few! All of the aforementioned reveal in their own words how much Steve Reeves' films and his incomparable physique have inspired them. If that weren't enough, even the late Sir Winston Churchill wrote in his autobiography that Steve Reeves was one of his two favorite film personalities — the other being John Wayne!

In terms of genetics, Steve Reeves possessed, in a word, "everything." Long, full muscle bellies in every muscle group; perfect proportions; unmatched symmetry; incredible lines and crowning it all was, perhaps, the most handsome face ever seen on stage or screen. Many say that in the sport of bodybuilding, having favorable genetics is akin to being born with a silver spoon in your mouth. Such is the degree of competitive leverage afforded by heredity. If this analogy is true, then Steve Reeves cannot be said to have a silver spoon in his mouth — hell, he had the whole damn cutlery store!

Not that he didn't have to work hard to develop "the greatest physique in the world" (a tag that has justifiably endured to this day), because he was and in fact remains the greatest and one of the most innovative bodybuilders of all time. When phenomenal genetics are married to proper training methodology, the end result — as Steve Reeves proved — is out and out perfection, or at least, as near to it as humanity has ever seen.

Moore's book also contained an interesting anecdote from famed Hollywood artist Ken Kendall, who had Reeves pose in his studio for a series of sketches and a bronze bust during the early 1950s. Kendall had sculpted busts of many of Hollywood's biggest stars, Marlon Brando and James Dean among them. One day, so the story goes, James Dean arrived at Kendall's studio in preparation to be sculpted. Dean, a longtime Brando fan, was admiring the work Kendall had done on the bronze bust of the famed "method" actor, when Kendall beckoned him to the rear of the studio.

"I pointed out the tableau of Reeves' zodiac etchings I had created," recalled Kendall. "Dean was familiar with them, and I could tell through his attitude that he certainly knew who Steve Reeves was and admired him very much. When I showed him a bust of Reeves that I had in progress, he remarked, "That is great!" When Kendall asked Dean if he knew who it was, the reply from the famed *Rebel Without A Cause* was instant: "It's the one and only Steve Reeves!"

With this same sense of awe and respect, I'm proud to count "the one and only" Steve Reeves as one of my close acquaintances, and I'm both delighted and honored that he chose Little-Wolff Books to be the publisher of his long-awaited book on *Building The Classic Physique — the Natural Way*.

— John Little

PREFACE

Whatever happened to a time when people worked hard for what they got? A time when folks understood that short-term gain more often than not leads to long-term pain. It seems today's society, especially many of the athletes, live and die by the creed, "I want it all, and I want it now!"— even if it means resorting to pills, tablets or injections to do it.

Fortunately, Steve Reeves was never such a man. Always one who believed that the sweat on the brow determined the quality and result of the effort, Steve Reeves carved an indelible mark in the history of bodybuilding as builder of the greatest natural physique of all time.

Sure, others have been bigger and stronger, but none better. Steve Reeves built his body at a time when bodybuilding drugs were unknown. Every one of his training methods was learned empirically — through trial and error — and for a natural physique. The way Steve transformed his body in such a short period of time was proof then, and even more so today, of what you can do if you have the best plan and strategies. This book, *Building the Classic Physique - the Natural Way*, will give you that plan and those strategies.

As much as we'd like, none of us will have a body exactly like Steve Reeves'. We are each genetically endowed with a body type and structure that is uniquely our own. Any book that promises you that you can change your inherent genetic structure is simply not giving it to you straight.

What this book will do is give you a lifetime of priceless experience that people just like you have been waiting for, and this is how to build your greatest body possible and do it naturally. You'll be amazed at how quickly this book will change your life.

There will never be another Steve Reeves. His image of movie star and physique legend continues to burn indelibly in our minds. Both my good friend, John Little, and I consider it an honor and a blessing that Steve Reeves asked us to be a part of this legacy of his life. We know you'll be blessed too.

Think of this book as a personal gift to you from Steve. For that's exactly how he wants it to be. Read his words. Embrace them. Learn from them. Most of all, apply them to your life today. Your life will never be the same. To your happiness and great success!

— **Bob Wolff, Ph.D.**

Foreword

At the close of World War II, I remember visiting Jack LaLanne's gym in the San Francisco Bay area, where I was enthusiastically shown a physique photo of a young guy they said was soon to return home from military duty in the Pacific. They guessed he was only 16 years old when the picture was taken. The structure and proportions on one so young, and the name Steve Reeves, were unforgettable.

One sunny day, some time later at Santa Monica's Muscle Beach, the epicenter of body culture during that era, a fully-dressed figure strolled out on the sand, looked around unassumingly, then casually stripped to his briefs. We observers were awestruck. I knew immediately this was that youngster in that photo come to life. The muscularity, proportions and lines seemed almost unreal, something from another time and space. The rest is history.

After winning major physique titles, Steve Reeves spent nearly two decades starring in European movies and became the world's leading motion picture actor of the times. Injuries caused by the tough demands of his *Hercules* roles forced him to retire. He settled on his ranch in Southern California, where he raised Morgan horses and became a mythical figure to the emerging generation of bodybuilders. In the late 1980s, the clamor for information on Reeves reached *Muscle and Fitness* magazine, for which I did a lengthy biography that once again brought the great Reeves' physique to public attention.

Until I did that story, I hadn't seen Steve for more than 30 years. Yet, I had never forgotten my early impressions of him. Those early musclemen of Southern California were delighted to have Steve among them. He was personable and fun-loving, and took his magnificent looks in stride. Even back then, he knew a lot about diet, and when he spoke, we listened. His mother, a nutritionist, had taught him well.

He enjoyed his perfection and shared it in fun with us by flexing his massive forearm or showing us his perfect teeth, cavity-free. He was unable to pull up his 18-inch pants cuff past his relaxed calf muscle. We once measured his shoulder width — tip to tip — at 23 and-a-half inches. Women, both young and old, followed him at the beach.

If something is perfect, it can't be more perfect. Yet Steve enhanced his natural endowments with muscle. He trained his own way, and never followed anyone. He knew exactly how he wanted to look. He eschewed training for sheer strength but rightly claimed he could get as strong as he wished.

Call it an epiphany, the appearance — no, its descent to earth — of the Reeves physique many years ago set an irreplaceable standard in bodybuilding and has inspired millions. It was great fun to have been part of its presence.

— **Armand Tanny, Senior Writer,** *Muscle and Fitness Magazine,* **Woodland Hills, California**

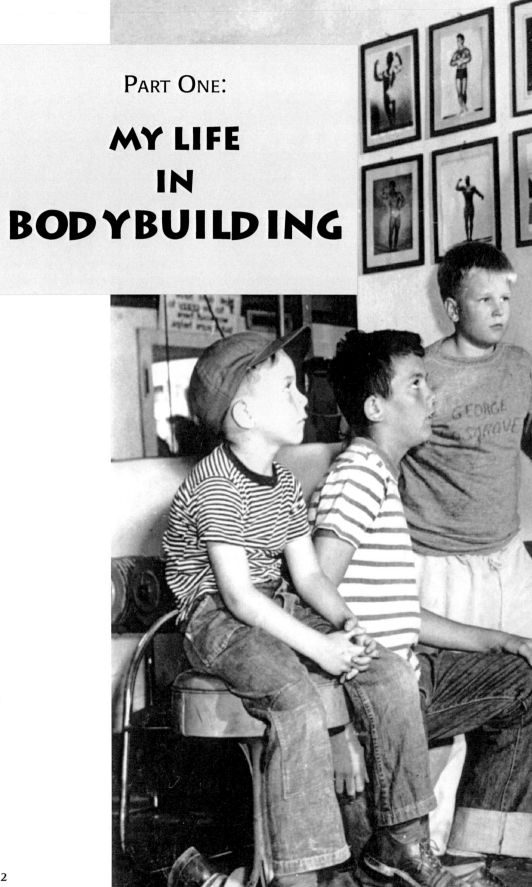

PART ONE:
MY LIFE IN BODYBUILDING

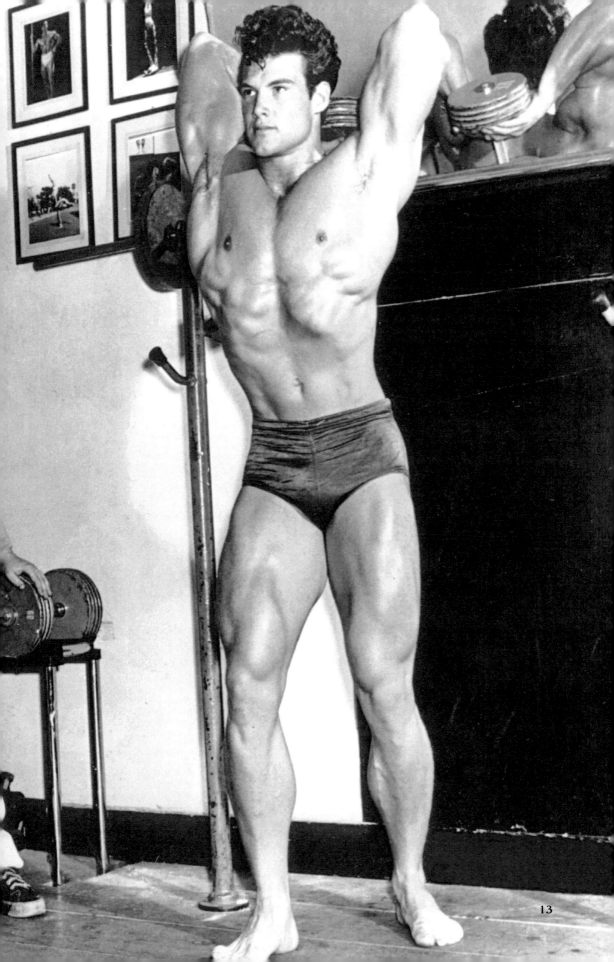

Chapter 1:
On the Shoulders of Giants

I suppose my story begins like that of most others — with those that went before me. My lineage is a combination of Irish, Welsh, German and English. On my mother's side, my great grandfather, Boyce, was a tailor by trade and came to America from England, settling with his wife in a town in Ohio. Later, his son Stephen Boyce moved from Ohio to Montana and eventually built a hotel and purchased a cattle and sheep ranch in the community of Scobey, Montana. In time, Stephen Boyce married and had six sons and a daughter, Golden Boyce — the lady that would eventually become my mother.

On the Reeves side of the family, my great grandfather was Manasseh Reeves, who was a veteran of the Civil War, fighting under General Sherman's command. Manasseh's son would, in time, become my paternal grandfather, Sylvester Reeves. Sylvester was born in Minnesota, but moved to Montana at some point during his youth. He had tremendous genetics, standing 6-foot-4-inches and weighing a hard 240 pounds. Eventually, he met and married Jessie Day, who in time gave him four sons: Ted, Claude, Lester and Archie. Unfortunately, problems arose in the marriage and Sylvester and Jessie Reeves divorced while the children were still quite young. Jesse eventually remarried to a man named Jack W. Peters.

Jack Peters and Jessie came to Scobey in 1914 and filed their homestead in that town the following year. Jessie took a job in a local restaurant to help out the family, while the boys Ted, Claude and Lester (sadly, Archie passed away prior to his 21st birthday), attended Scobey High School. Claude enlisted in the Army in World War I and did not return to Scobey until he was asked to come back and help out on the ranch. Ted was given a scholarship to the University of California at Berkeley but on the way to campus met a young lady named Geneva, in Portland, Oregon — and never made it to California.

In the meantime, Jack Peters, Jessie Reeves Peters and Jessie's son, Lester, leased land for a ranch near Richland, Montana. Lester did carpentry and contracting work, in addition to helping out on the ranch. Lester courted Golden Boyce, a neighbor in Scobey, and the two were considered by the people in Daniels County to be the most attractive couple of the time.

Lester had obviously inherited his father Sylvester's genetics, standing 6-foot-1-inch and checking in at a rock-solid 200 pounds. He had broad shoulders and was a tremendously fit individual. On April 3, 1924 Lester married "Goldie" (who was a beautiful person — both physically and emotionally) in a simple ceremony in Scobey. Less than two years later, they would become my parents.

I was born on January 21, 1926, in the home of my uncle, Stephen Boyce Jr., in Glasgow, Montana, the only child of Lester and Goldie Reeves. In retrospect, I believe that I inherited much of my genetics for bodybuilding from my father, Lester, because when I was six months old, my mother entered me in my first contest in which I was awarded first place in the "Healthiest Baby in Daniels County."

These were good times in a short-lived marriage for my parents. Tragedy struck our home in October of 1927 when my father was killed in a freak farming accident. He had been in the fields watching the harvesting operation and got to talking to one of the hands. At that moment, one of the workers got his pitchfork caught in the belts of the thresher and — without warning — the pitchfork was yanked from the worker's hands and soared back towards my dad. It pierced his intestine and, although he was immediately rushed to a local doctor in Scobey, who quickly administered medical treatment, infection quickly set in and, despite taking him by train to the nearest hospital (which was 250 miles away in Minot, North Dakota), within 48 hours, my father was dead. I was just 20 months old at the time. I remember my mother telling me years later that, at my father's funeral, a small boy about six years of age looked up sadly at his mother and asked, "I wonder what will ever become of Lester's son?"

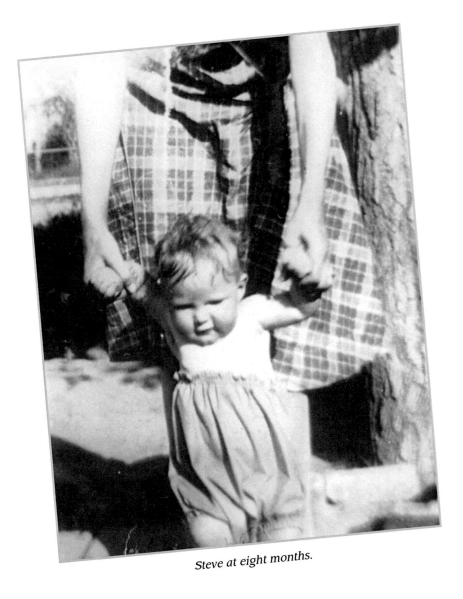

Steve at eight months.

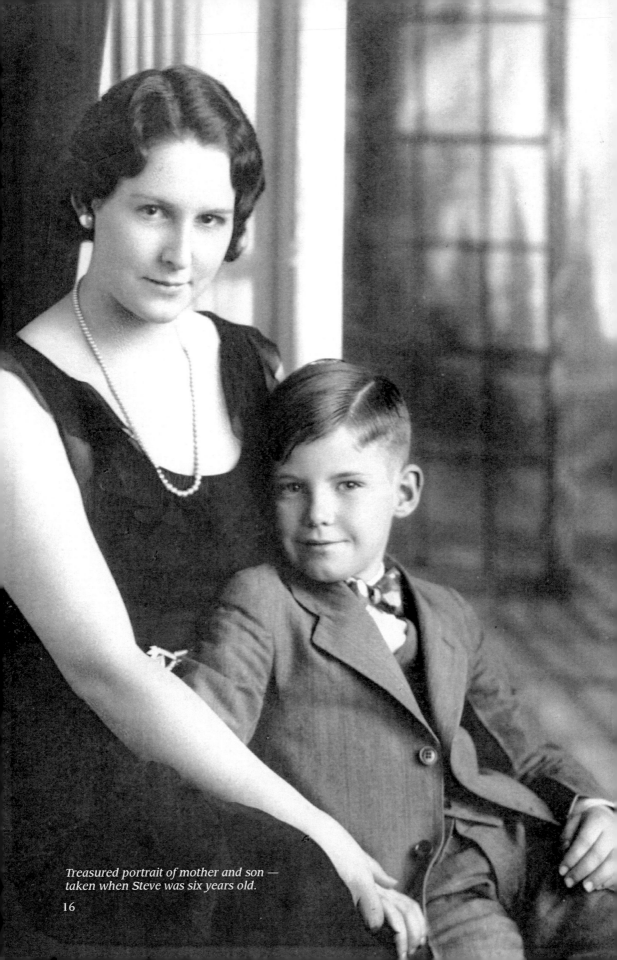

Treasured portrait of mother and son — taken when Steve was six years old.

Chapter 2:
Moving Forward

After the passing of my dad, my mother did the best she could. Times were tough for her, and after enduring much hardship, she packed me up with all of our belongings and headed for Scobey, where her family lived on a ranch. My memories of that ranch are still vivid today. I thoroughly took to ranch living — which resulted in a love of ranching that I enjoy to this day. I took to horseback riding at three years of age. My favorite mount was a kindly old horse named Old Dan. I used to ride Dan into the pasture every morning. When my mother wanted to check in on me or to call me back for lunch, she would ring a loud, clanking bell and, at that sound, Old Dan would slowly plod his way back to the ranch house with me on his back and would receive a handful of grain as his reward.

During the time my mother lived with her family on the ranch, she actively sought employment throughout Scobey. Unfortunately, there just weren't any jobs at that time but, fortunately, some of mom's friends from church pooled their funds when they got wind of her plight, and gave her the money she needed to move to Great Falls, Montana (approximately 380 miles southwest of Scobey) where jobs were more plentiful. Shortly after arriving in Great Falls, my mom took a job as a cook at the Rainbow Hotel.

My mother and I moved into a little place in town that was close to her work. In a short time, she gained a reputation as an outstanding cook and was offered a position as the personal cook for Dr. Porter, who was at that time one of Great Falls' most prominent physicians. Dr. Porter had room for a single live-in employee, but no accommodations for a child. Not wanting to pass up the opportunity or the money offered by Dr. Porter, my mother sought out a boarding school for me. She settled on the Montana Deaconess School — a religious boarding school. It was a difficult decision for my mother, as the school was more than 90 miles from Great Falls. Nevertheless, after a thorough inspection of the grounds and facilities, I found myself enrolled in the Montana Deaconess school. Although I missed my mother a lot — over the next three years, I only got to see her once a month, and sometimes during the summer months — the change was somewhat refreshing.

At school there was a certain amount of independence and the chance to be competitive and active with other children of the same age. I recall entering a Bible contest at the school when I was six years old. To win I had to recite from memory 10 pages of scripture. The prize was a beautiful Bible. I won the contest and still have that Bible. And one year later, I got my first taste of show business by winning $5.00 for reciting a poem.

My favorite times, however, were when I was able to get together with my mother and cousins on my uncle's ranch during the warm summer months. I remember once when I was riding into the pasture in search of adventure with my twin cousins Violet and Viola. We dismounted from one of the ranch horses and began playing in the grassy meadow when all of a sudden, a rather large bull appeared. It snorted at us and began pawing the ground. I knew it was going to charge us. Sensing danger immediately, I bolted for the girls just as the bull began its charge. I quickly grabbed each of the girls around their waists and hoisted them onto the back of the horse. Then I quickly jumped up onto the horse myself and we were off before the bull could even break into a full run!

Another time riding wasn't quite as exciting, however. I was riding one of my favorite horses, a mare named Smokie. For some reason, Smokie got spooked and reared up, falling over backwards — on top of me! I struggled to get the horse off of me and could feel my ribs breaking with each move I made. It took me over 10 minutes to get Smokie off me, and then I had to climb back on the horse and ride it to the ranch — broken ribs and all.

One day on the way home from school, I was hit by a car as I was walking back to my mom's house. I misjudged the speed of an oncoming car as I was crossing the street. Wham! It happened so fast I didn't know that I'd been hit — until I realized that I was hanging on to the front bumper and being dragged along the asphalt. The car came to a screeching halt about 50 yards later and the driver, a very distraught lady, rushed to the front of the vehicle where I was still holding on.

"Are you all right?" she asked. "Yes, I'm fine," I replied, still not completely sure what had just happened to me. "Let me take you to your home," she said, "Where do you live?" I couldn't tell her because I didn't want my mother to find out and scold me for foolishly running out in front of a car. Instead, I picked myself up, brushed off my clothes and walked back to where the car first hit me — with sufficient force to rip my shoe from my foot. I picked it up, put it on and walked home. I was absolutely filthy from being dragged under the car but, surprisingly, I suffered absolutely no injuries whatsoever.

When I got home, my mother took one look at me and said, "What happened to you?"

"Oh, I was playing with this dirty, old stick," I replied (where I pulled this explanation out of, I still haven't a clue!). Anyway she bought it (I told her the truth — but years later you understand).

While I learned to dodge traffic a little more precisely after that experience, the one hit I had absolutely no defense for (and neither did anyone else), was the Montana earthquake of 1935. In fact, two earthquakes hit; the first on October 3, and the second on October 12, measuring 5.0 and 7.0 respectively. The second one really shook up the Deaconess Boarding School. As it hit in the morning, all of us were sleeping in our beds. My dormitory was on the third floor of the brick school building and, after the quake hit, everyone went running outside for safety. Once outside the teachers could account for all of the students — except yours truly. After calling my name repeatedly and looking everywhere outside for me, two men decided to search the dorm.

The old brick building that housed the dormitory had suffered a major hit. Some of the exterior walls had collapsed and debris was everywhere. The electrical power was out but the two men made their way to what used to be my room. The outside wall of the room was gone and they found my bed — with me still sleeping in it — hanging out about a foot through the opening and covered with fallen bricks. (Hey, I've always been a sound sleeper, what can I say?) They woke me gently, not wanting me to step out of bed — with the wall missing, I would have fallen three stories!

The school suffered a total loss and had to be rebuilt. When the earth finally settled down, Montana had experienced no less than 1,346 aftershocks from the '35 quake.

Chapter 3:
Go West, Young Man

In the early part of 1936, one of my mother's closest friends, a lady named Frances Chamberlain, moved to Oak Knoll, a community in Oakland, California. My mother had known Frances since her late teens. When Frances told her that there were plenty of employment opportunities for her in Northern California, my mother had no reason to doubt her and decided to make the move. It was soon going to be summer and she knew she would have plenty of time to prepare for the move West.

In June of that year, after school was out, I received an invitation to spend a few weeks of summer with the Hall family at their cabin on the Smith River in Montana. The Halls were my old family friends. I was ten years old at the time and spent my last Montana summer with the Halls' six children at their family cabin.

The cabin was rustic, yet comfortable — and it could only be reached by hiking down the side of an incredibly steep hill. I noticed right away that trying to control my speed coming down this hill was great exercise for my quadriceps. When Vernon, the eldest of the Hall children, would return from town with the groceries, he would park his car at the top of the hill and we'd all climb that hill, grab up an armful of grocery bags and then — with the added resistance — carefully negotiate that steep hill down to the cabin. It usually took several trips to get all of the food and supplies, and I eventually ended up loading several bags at a time in a backpack. In fact, it was probably these backpack expeditions that first awakened in me a sense of physical well-being from exercise.

That summer was really enjoyable and allowed me to be extremely physically active, which is the ideal tonic for restless children. Every day I was either hiking, swimming, fishing or carrying firewood. I remember that Vernon would split the logs with a huge ax and I'd marvel at his physique. When he would take off his shirt and swing that ax his muscles flexed with every move. I remember that Vernon was the first person whose physique had truly impressed me. I told him, "Boy, I wish I had arms like yours!" Vernon just smiled at me and said, "Maybe by the next time you see me, you will." It was the last time I would ever see Vernon, but I've never forgotten him — nor his influence.

The very next day my mother showed up and scooped me up from the Halls to take me on a vacation with her. We were off to see the World Exposition of 1936, which was being held in San Diego.

After the visiting the World Exposition, my mother and I continued on to Oakland, where I would spend the next eight years of my life. The job situation in Oakland was not quite as rosy as my mother had hoped. The best job available was as a cook for a wealthy family in Napa, which is located in California's picturesque wine country. Once again, the employers had living quarters for her — but not for a child. Fortunately, my mother had some close friends, the Chamberlains, and they offered to have me move in with them — which I did, for the next three years.

I attended elementary school in Oak Knoll and made several friends there. My friends and I loved to collect lead bullets that we found at an abandoned military target range. We'd dig the bullets out of the hills and melt them down, pour the molten lead into a mold to create things like ornaments in the shapes of Christmas trees and other holiday objects.

There were horses nearby —which I loved — and it didn't take me long to discover where the horse stables were located. During the summers I would ride the horses and spend hours watching the trainers work with and groom them.

Occasionally, my friends and I would take a half-hour bus ride to the movie house to catch the latest westerns. I earned money for these movie trips by delivering the Sunday newspaper on my bicycle.

My bicycle riding laid the foundation for my future leg development. When I was 12 years old, I rode my bicycle over the big hill between Oak Knoll and east Oakland so that I could visit with my friends. I would pedal my bike two miles up the hill and two miles down. Many of my friends walked their bikes up the hill. But I always loved a challenge, so I would tell myself, "I will make it all the way to the top, or I will break a chain trying, or be forced to stop from pure exhaustion."

I broke many chains (long before I did so in films like Hercules!) in my quest to make it over that hill. After a couple years of pedaling up and down the hill, it became routine for me. My legs actually developed — particularly my calves — quite quickly.

While I was attending Frick Junior High School, my mother met a gentleman named Earl Maylone through the Chamberlains. Earl worked as an installer/repairman for the telephone company. They were married in 1939 and I moved with them to their new home on 76 Avenue in East Oakland. The house was within the school district and I was able to complete my years at Frick.

By the time I turned 13, I had increased my newspaper route from Sundays only to seven days a week. This gave me more spending money for entertainment, which I often spent on movies. In my last year of junior high school, I was able to do many things, most importantly of which was getting to again live with my mother and getting acquainted with my stepfather. I was also developing something of a reputation for myself as being the undisputed king of arm-wrestling among my friends.

Chapter 4: I Discover Bodybuilding

One day while I was delivering newspapers along my route, I met a boy named Joe Gambina. Joe and I were about the same age (16 years) and we soon began talking. Feeling tremendously confident, I introduced the subject of arm wrestling and how I was the best at it in my school. Joe said he was a "pretty good" arm wrestler himself. Shortly thereafter, our arms were locked and a match was on. It ended as quickly as it started — whomp! — with my arm pinned to the table!

I was dumbfounded, particularly since I was already much bigger than Joe, who stood only 5-foot-5-inches and weighed maybe 140 pounds. Still in disbelief, I told Joe that we'd lock arms again when I didn't have so many newspapers to deliver.

As I hopped back on my bike and pedaled it down the street, I couldn't get over the fact that this guy had beaten me. I kept asking myself over and over, "How did I lose to this guy — when he's so much smaller than I am?" I would find out the answer a few weeks later.

I kept in touch with Joe, and when he told me that he had a bicycle rack for sale, I hurried over to his house later to pick it up. When I knocked on his door, Joe's sister answered and informed me that Joe wasn't in the house, but was "out back in the garage — working out." I stared at her and asked, "Working out? What's that?" She just pointed toward the garage and said, "You'd better go and see for yourself."

When I entered the garage, there was Joe lifting weights. I asked what the heck he was doing. Joe simply finished his set, walked over to a table where a magazine had been placed, picked it up and handed me the copy of *Strength and Health Magazine*, one of the first periodicals dedicated to bodybuilding and strength training.

On the front cover was a photo of a very well-developed man named John Grimek. Grimek looked incredible to me! His arms were magnificent and his legs were equally as impressive. I'd never seen anything like this before in my life. In fact, I didn't even know it was possible for a human being to look like that! Excitedly, I started

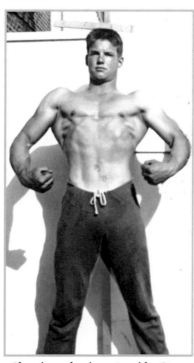

Showing a beginner's pride, Steve poses at sixteen years of age.

speaking with Joe about bodybuilding and looked through a few more of his bodybuilding magazines. I knew, at the instant I first saw that shot of Grimek, that this was how I wanted to be built. I looked Joe square in the eye and asked, "Can we work out together?"

Joe nodded quickly in agreement, "Sure," he said, and them added, "and I'll only charge you 50 cents a workout."

For the next several weeks Joe and I worked on creating bodybuilding routines.

By this point, I'd done some reading on my own and better understood what I was doing. I saved up my newspaper money and purchased a 200 pound set of used weights that I found in a classified ad. Soon my training venue switched from Joe's garage to my own, and my parents didn't seem to mind that I'd converted part of their garage into my own personal "gym."

At this time I was six feet tall but weighed a mere 156 pounds stripped. I began from these humble beginnings to record my first workout schedule of exercises, reps and weight on one

My First Workout Schedule

Exercise	Sets	Reps	Weight
Warm up: (Dumbbell Swings)	1	20	10 pounds
Clean	1	10	60 pounds
Military Press	1	10	60 pounds
Supine Press	1	10	70 pounds
Rowing	1	10	60 pounds
Reverse Curl	1	10	30 pounds
Regular Curl	1	10	40 pounds
Squats	1	10	100 pounds
Breathing Dumbbell Pullover	1	10	20-pound dumbbells
Good Mornings	1	10	60 pounds
Breathing Lateral Raise	1	10	10-pound dumbbells

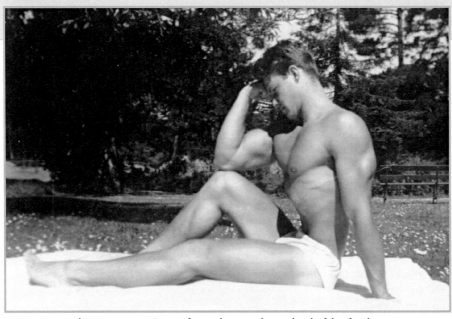

In just one year, Steve shows impressive gains in his physique.

of the interior garage walls in white chalk. Interestingly enough, that garage wall workout was recently discovered perfectly in tact by my friend, George Helmer (see appendix at the back of this book). I recall that I used as much weight as I could handle for each exercise in perfect form (a practice I continued all through my championship years right up until present day) and this initial training program included only one set of each exercise.

It was a great beginner's workout and served to prepare my body for the more demanding training I would later engage in. I always took my workouts in stride and never tried to overload my body with too much exercise at a time when my system needed most of its energy for growing and for normal development.

As soon as I was able to complete 12 repetitions in perfect form, I would increase the resistance I was using by five pounds and would drop back to 10 repetitions once more.

I followed this program for the first three months of my bodybuilding career after which I used the same exercises, the same system of increasing poundages and the same number of reps, but I did two sets of each exercise instead of one. Soon, my body weight was up to 163 pounds — it felt incredible!

I attended Oakland's Castlemont High School from 1941 to 1944. Castlemont included sophomore through senior grade levels. I did very well in athletics during my sophomore year and the football coach always kept a close watch on the new sophomores in diligent search of the next generation of potential gridiron heroes.

After watching me for several days, the coach asked if I would like to play defensive guard for the school team — this happened just two months after I began working out on my first program! I'd already gained considerable muscle mass and strength at that point. Although I was flattered by the invitation, I told the coach I wanted to wait until the next year to join the team.

I wanted more time to gain the size I felt I would need to be a better defensive guard. When the following year came, my high school offered a program where you could go to school half a day and work half a day to help the war effort and still get full credit. So I never did get to play football.

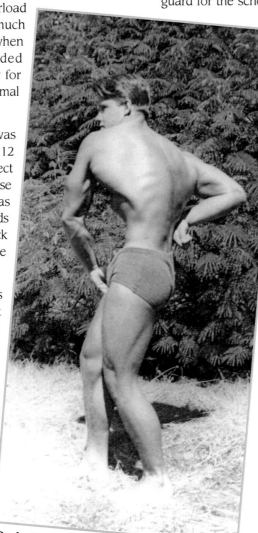

Back shot of the seventeen-year-old Reeves.

Chapter 5: Enter Ed Yarick

Ed Yarick was a noted bodybuilding coach with a gym in Oakland. Ed had been featured in many of the muscle magazines that were popular at the time and, after having spent a couple of months training in my garage and achieving a solid base level of strength and size, I learned of Ed's gym. I stopped by one afternoon and Ed explained his training methods and nutritional theories to me. I liked what I heard and decided it was time to start training at a "real" gym, instead of my garage — and thus began a lifelong friendship with Ed Yarick and his family.

One of the first programs that I worked out on under Ed's supervision was the following:

My Second Workout Schedule

Exercise	Sets	Reps	Weight
Dumbbell Swings (warm up)	3	15-20	moderate
Upright Rowing	3	8-12	as much as possible
Supine Press (Bench Press)	3	8-12	as much as possible
One-Arm Dumbbell Rows	3	8-12	as much as possible
Dumbbell Laterals	3	8-12	as much as possible
Incline Presses	3	8-12	decreasing weight
Triceps Pushdowns	3	8-12	as much as possible
Barbell Curls	3	8-12	as much as possible
Seated Dumbbell Curls	3	8-12	as much as possible
Full Squats	3	8-12	as much as possible
(Supersetted with) Pullovers	3	8-12	as much as possible
Breathing Squats	1	20	as much as possible
(Supersetted with) Breathing Pullovers	1	20	as much as possible
Deadlifts	2	8-12	as much as possible
Good Mornings	2	8-12	as much as possible

I always performed my squats with a two or three inch board under my heels. I've found this to be the best way to perform full squats. I came to this conclusion on my own, simply because I used to do my squats in high-heeled field boots and found that the exercise was of far greater value when done in this manner. This last system of training I followed for eight months (with only some slight modifications), thereby rounding out my first year of training with weights.

I used to perform an exercise — not seen much these days but highly effective nonetheless — at Yarick's called "Breathing Squats." This required you to select a weight that you could squat with about 20 times and do five heavy breaths in between each squat. As soon as you put the bar back on the rack, you were to do Breathing Pullovers which, we were told, would help to increase the size of the rib box and thus, create a far more dramatic contrast between our chest and waist.

When I first started at Ed Yarick's Gym and wanted to get a really good basic build, he had me perform these special exercises that really emphasized breathing. I would inhale and exhale as much as I could in-between reps — really deep breaths — and then I would hold the last breath and do a full squat. It's very demanding because my chest would be just heaving at the completion of the set and then I'd rush over to do a set of Breathing Pullovers. These required a lighter weight, but the focus was on expanding the rib box and getting a good stretch and contraction.

I was learning more and more about training and nutrition all the time, and under Ed's watchful eye, I gained 30 pounds of solid muscle in just four months of training at his gym. The first month my bodyweight stayed at 163 pounds but my physique noticeably hardened up. The following month I went up to 173 pound; the next month I was at 183 pounds; and the next month, I was 193 pounds. In fact, after just four months of focused, intense training, Yarick told me that I was the best-built guy at the gym — and there were guys working out there who had been training for well over three years. However, it took me another year to get from 193 to 203 pounds, utilizing the "Classic Physique" routine outlined in Part Two of this book.

In the summer following my sophomore year, I was 16 years old and loading pallets at the Del Monte cannery in Oakland. The next year I worked at the Army Quartermaster Supply Depot. I loaded railroad cars and trucks with war supplies. By that time, World War II was in full swing and Castlemont High School was put on half-day sessions. I attended my classes in the morning and continued to work at the Depot in the afternoon. The students took mandatory classes and received credit for afternoon work.

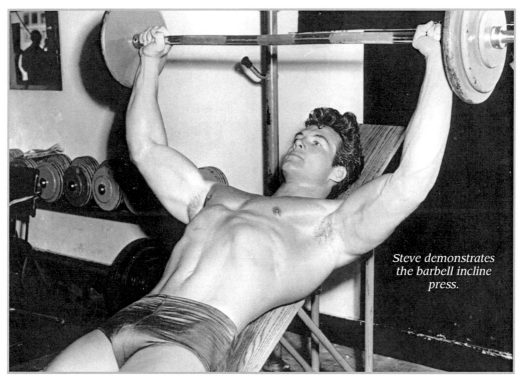

Steve demonstrates the barbell incline press.

During my junior year, I attended high school from 8:00 a.m. to 12:00 p.m., then walked to my job at the Depot where I worked from 1:00 p.m. to 5:00 p.m. Then three days a week headed for Ed's gym, where I worked out from 5:30 p.m. to 7:30 p.m. Since I spent so much of my time either working or working out, it left little time for the usual high school activities such as proms, parties or participating in extracurricular sports.

When I wasn't going to school, working or working out, I was collecting metal for use in the war effort. Residents and businesses would set out their scrap or discarded metal at the curb for pick- up. One day while I was picking up war metal, I found a set of bodybuilding wall pulleys in the curb pickup. I really wanted them, although I knew they were supposed to go toward the war effort. But I knew they could help me a lot in my quest to build a classic physique. I took the pulleys but — in fairness — replaced them with an equal amount of iron I gathered from my neighbors and my own home. Since Ed had only one set of pulleys in his gym, I gave him my set and the two of us immediately installed them across from the other set. These proved to be the first-ever set of crossover pulleys in the Oakland area and we used them all the time.

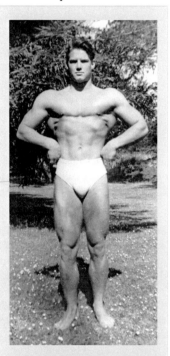

My body began to fill out quickly and proportionately. Soon I was the talk of the school. Granted, training with weights was not a popular notion to subscribe to in those days. In high school, the coaches wouldn't let their football players swim because it would make their players' muscles "too soft." They wouldn't let their players lift weights or ride a bicycle because doing so was believed to make one's muscles "too tight." So weight lifting, cycling and swimming were banned for any athlete who wanted to play football or any other athletic event in those days! In fact, it was the complete opposite of what the enlightened coaches of today believe.

During the winter months, I enjoyed skating at the local Oakland ice rink. On one occasion I was at the rink with Ed and his wife, Alice and some of our friends from Ed's gym. We noticed a guy in a skintight T-shirt on the ice who was showing off and just acting obnoxious. Ed wanted to subtlety put the guy in his place, so he had my friends put up a five dollar bet that I wouldn't take off my baggy wool sweater and skate in front of the guy, just to see the look on his face when a real bodybuilder came by.

When I heard there was five bucks in it for me, my sweater was off! I wasn't completely insane, mind you, for I had on a bright red skintight T-shirt underneath that was tapered to reveal my muscles to their fullest. I glided onto the ice and passed by the obnoxious guy without even a glance back at him. According to my friends, the guy stood there dumbfounded and nearly lost his balance before heading quickly toward the nearest exit! I casually skated back to the group, grabbed my five dollars and quickly put on my sweater!

By graduation, I was very pleased with my rate of progress since starting bodybuilding, and my measurements were now:

Weight:	203 pounds
Height:	6' 1"
Neck:	17¼"
Chest:	47½"
Waist:	29"
Biceps:	17¼"
Hips:	37"
Thigh:	24½"
Calf:	17¼"

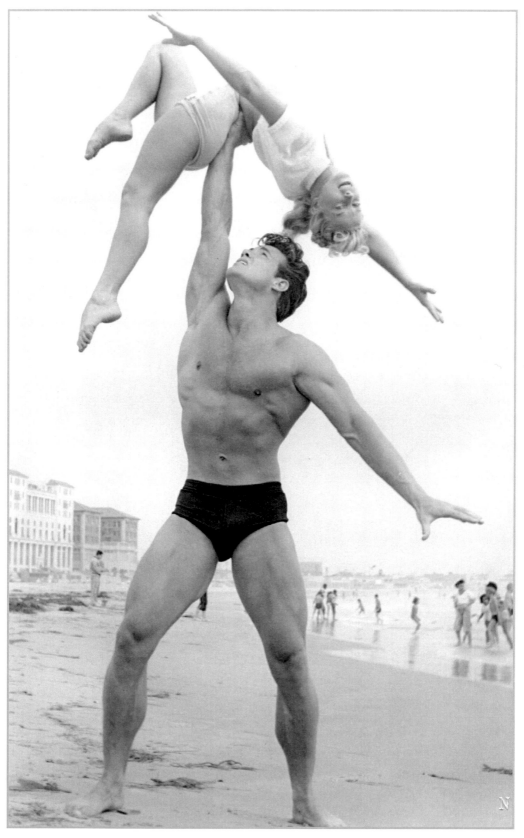

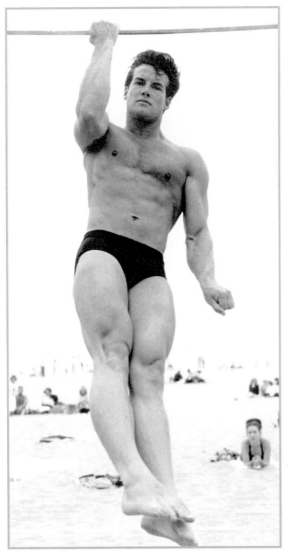

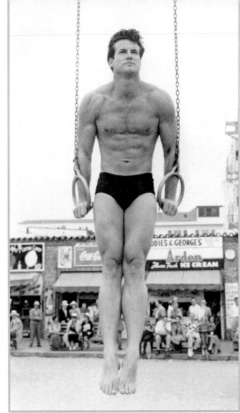

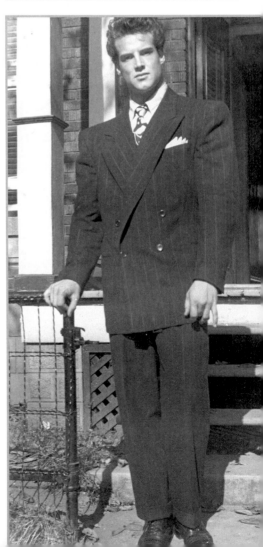

During that summer between high school and the armed forces, Steve discovered Muscle Beach in Santa Monica and would return to live there. Previous page and above: Steve performs gymnastic stunts, the one-arm chin-up and a routine on the rings.

Right: After winning the 1947 Mr. America, Steve visits photographer Tony Lanza in Montreal, Canada.

Upper left and lower portion of opposite page: In preparation for the 1948 Mr. World (title awarded him in Cannes, France), Steve works out on the French Riviera.

Upper right, opposite page: Steve braves chilly weather in London doing publicity shots for the 1950 Mr. Universe contest.

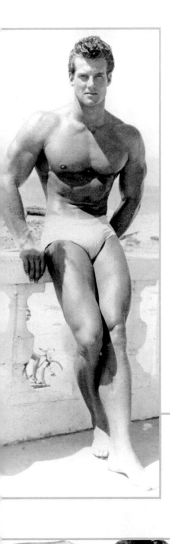
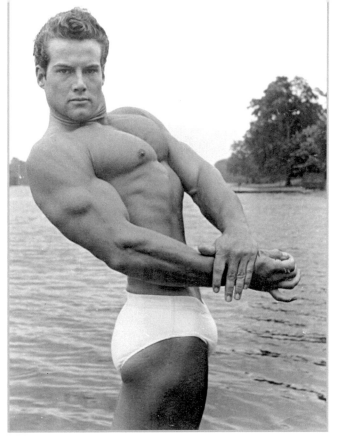
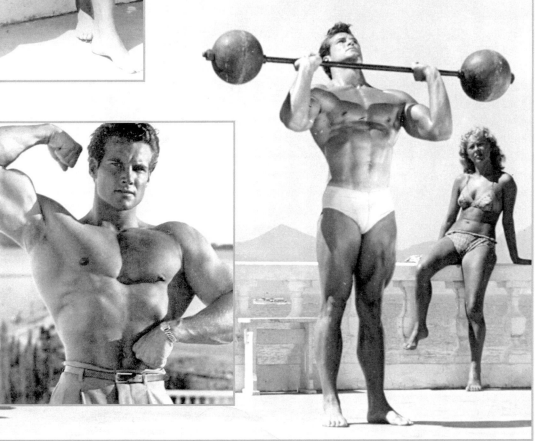

Chapter 6: Life in the Service

After two years of bodybuilding, I was inducted into the Army. I was stationed in the States for three months of basic training and then shipped to the Philippines, and was eventually assigned to the 25th Combat Division of the Infantry as a replacement.

Waiting for placement, I looked around for something to exercise with. I ran across six one-gallon cans that had been filled with cement, and quickly affixed them to a bar so that I could use it as a makeshift barbell. I located a rope that had been discarded from a ship and used it for climbing, which gave my lats, delts, biceps and forearms a great workout. I also found an old anchor chain which I cut into eight-foot lengths. I attached these to the ends of my makeshift barbell and discovered that as I lifted the barbell higher, more and more links of the chain would be picked up by the barbell, which effectively increased the resistance that my muscles were contracting against. The higher the barbell was lifted, the more resistance I got. This very well may have been the forerunner of the "Variable Resistance Principle" used years later on the Universal and Nautilus exercise machines.

This equipment was okay, but I knew I would need more weight. One day while I was walking around in the jungle, a very slight Filipino man approached me and asked me if I'd like to buy a barbell set — you could have knocked me over with a feather! I ended up purchasing a 100-pound York Barbell set while in the jungles of the Philippines for 20 American dollars, and started working out with a fellow named Tony, until we were shipped out.

I discovered that, for a person of 203 pounds bodyweight, a 100-pound barbell set just wasn't heavy enough to get a productive workout using conventional methods. However, I learned a lot about training — and the importance of perfect exercise style — from training with that little barbell set. I discovered that it wasn't just the weight you were using, but how you used it that was the important factor in building muscle.

I kept records of particular exercises and which muscle groups were affected while

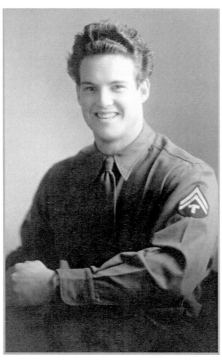
Steve in Manila —1945.

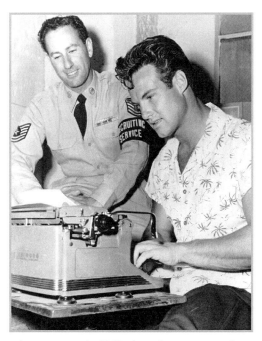

*Above: Steve dutifully does the paper work.
Below: "The Shape"*

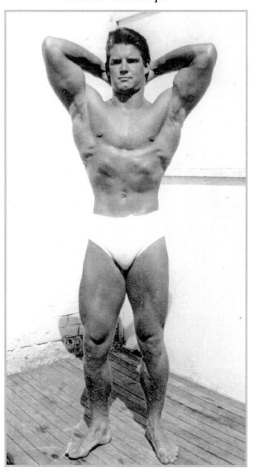

performing a particular exercise (I still have this log). When I was working out at Ed Yarick's gym, we would routinely squat upwards of 300 pounds but since I had only 100 pounds to work with in the Philippines, I had to make the most out of what I had.

I began to perform my reps slowly and with deep concentration, and would perform as many repetitions as I could. I found that not only did I get a great cardiovascular workout from doing my squats this way, but my leg gains were also very good. At the end of the time I trained in the Philippines, I was doing 100 reps in a row without pausing — with 100 pounds on my back (which was approximately half of my bodyweight) — in squats!

When I was finally shipped towards the front lines, I took my weights with me. Three of my buddies carried 25 pounds each, and we stored the bar along with rifles that were heading in the same direction. I earned the nickname "The Shape," from other members of my division (they later shortened it to simply "Shape"), and shortly thereafter, I was sent to the front lines, assigned to Company A of the 25th Division.

Our company was involved in the taking of Balete Pass, which exposed me to warfare and it's horrors for the first time. In order not to become devastated by the death and destruction I witnessed going on all around me, I would try and detach myself mentally from what was going on. I began to look at myself as an observer — not as a participant in the action. I saw men killed and soldiers carried out on stretchers on a daily basis.

One time, as I was moving from position to position along the front lines, I saw one man who was on a stretcher. As the attendants picked him up for transport, his leg fell off — right off the stretcher and on to the ground! Somebody casually bent down, picked it up and tossed it back on the stretcher. Another fellow was shot in the stomach and his intestines were actually hanging outside of his body. It was horrible, but I was able to remain calm by distancing myself from what was going on and by forming vivid mental images of myself being anywhere but where I was.

In June of 1945 I contracted malaria and had seven very severe attacks of it during the next seven months, which resulted in my weight dropping from 203 to 175 pounds. Before the malaria, my weight and measurements had remained the same as they were when I was inducted (which was a phenomenon I noted later on in my life when I was making movies — my muscles stayed with me and I would need only four to six weeks of solid training to build them back up to top form).

After two months of malaria I was transferred to the Quartermaster Corps, and in September of 1945 I was sent to Japan as part of the occupation troops. During my long illness, I had had no chance whatsoever to train with weights. And, sick as I was, had very little incentive. However, in Japan I began to feel like myself again. With the war now over and with a new lease on life, I decided to do something about my physique once more.

I found a Japanese interpreter who took me to a foundry. There I designed and gave instructions for construction of a 210-pound barbell set, for which I paid 100 American dollars.

I kept the weights under my bed in the barracks and then built an exercise bench which passed army inspections because it looked enough like an ironing board to fool the inspecting officers. Actually the bench was often used as an ironing board, so it proved to be a success both ways.

I also managed to acquire a mirror that I hung near my bed where I would train, allowing me a gym-like atmosphere right in the heart of Japan. I used this setup for my workouts the last eight months of my time in the service, and increased my bodyweight from 175 to 195 pounds. In September of 1946 I was finally able to return home.

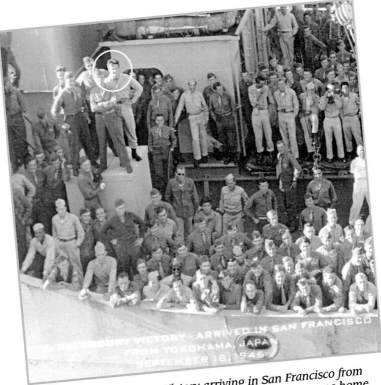

The H. M. Waterbury Victory arriving in San Francisco from Yokohama, Japan — September 18, 1946 — Steve came home.

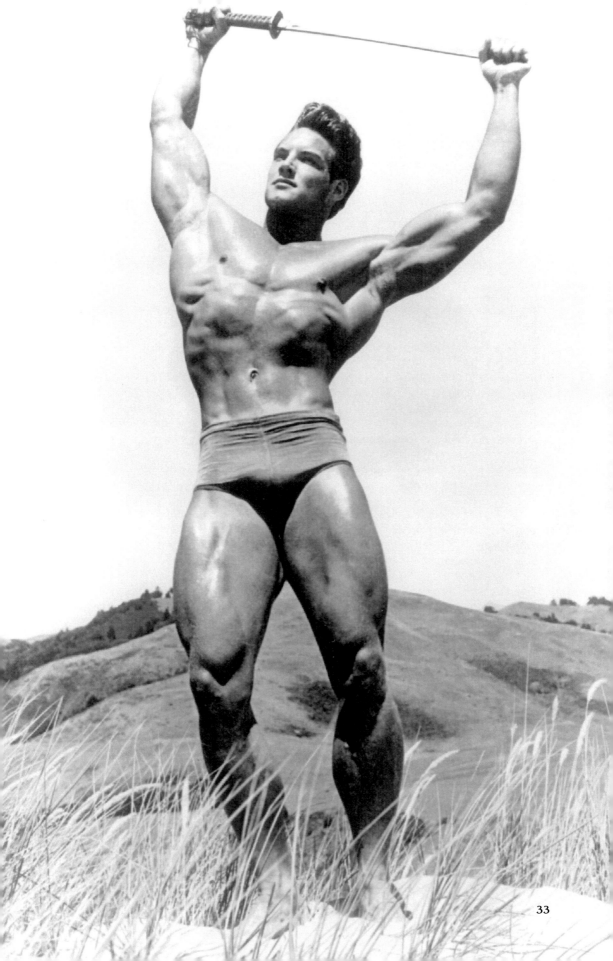

Chapter 7: My Bodybuilding Career Begins!

Home once more, I renewed my training with gusto at Ed Yarick's Gym using the Classic Physique program I developed (outlined in Part Two of this book) and within a few weeks I was back to 205 pounds! In December of 1946 I entered and won the Mr. Pacific Coast Contest in Portland, Oregon. Filled with confidence and optimism, I continued to train hard three days a week — and to gain more muscle. In May of 1947 I won the Mr. Western America title in Los Angeles.

While these titles were nice, I realized that they were only grist for the mill. The one title I wanted more than anything else was the Mr. America title — and when I finally won it in June of 1947, it was probably the proudest moment of my competitive career. The bodybuilding press of the day also seemed suitably impressed, causing one of the days top scribes, Gordon Venables, to write the following in Bob Hoffman's *Strength & Health* magazine:

"A thunderous approbation of hand clapping that gave way to cheers and whistles let the judges know in no uncertain terms their acceptance of Steve Reeves as Mr. America...You have to see this young man to really appreciate his build and good looks. Photos don't do him justice; he's twice as good looking as his pictures. It would be utter futility for me to try and describe in mere words his physique...'breathtaking' might give you some idea of the audience reaction...As readers will recall, I never did lean heavily to Mr. America contests when these events were in their embryonic stages. It was my contention that such shows were not for the real iron man. Now I've changed my opinion!...I believe a change has been wrought in the conception of the perfect male physique...Now we have a streamlined conception of the perfect masculine physique and Steve Reeves epitomizes that conception.

His tremendous breadth of shoulders and extreme slimness of waist are symbolic of the new physique. He exemplifies speed and grace rather than brute strength...I sincerely believe that if Eugene Sandow could have been called back from the Land of Shades to step upon the posing platform against Reeves, Sandow would have lost!"

While the accolades are always nice, my goal has always been to improve rather than to impress; to face tougher competition and evolve in my sport. To that end, I looked to the 1948 Mr. Universe contest, which was staged that year in London, England on August 23. I was 22 years old and was delighted to learn that at this contest I would be facing no less an adversary than John Grimek— the man whose picture on a magazine cover had first inspired me to pursue bodybuilding.

Months before the contest, the competitors were notified that they would be judged by height categories. Oscar Heidenstam's *Health & Strength* supplied further details in its July 15 edition:

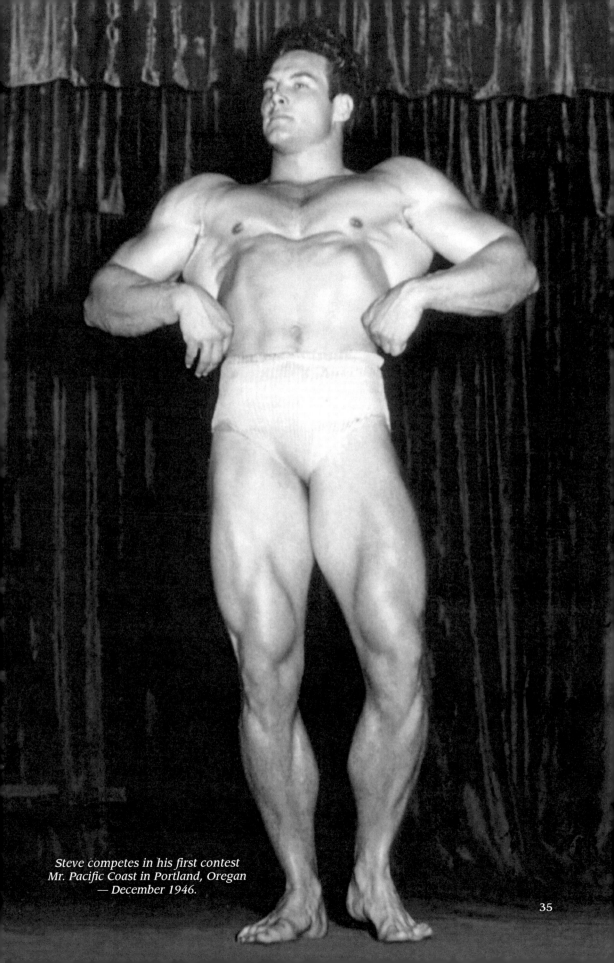

Steve competes in his first contest Mr. Pacific Coast in Portland, Oregan — December 1946.

"Judges will examine each class separately and choose the number of finalists to appear on stage. Each athlete will be allowed sufficient time to show his physique, posing ability and physical powers."

The judging panel included Bob Hoffman, publisher of Strength & Health and the head of the York Barbell Club of York, Pennsylvania; George Hackenschmidt of Germany; Tromp Van Deggelen of South Africa; photographer Arax of Paris; and British weightlifting authority George Walsh.

Among the leading contenders were the 1947 Mr. France, Andre Drapp; Mr. France runner-up, Juan Ferrero; Mahmoud Namdjou of Iran; and England's Oscar Heidenstam, publisher of Health & Strength and president of the National Amateur British Bodybuilder's Association (NABBA).

I wasn't prepared for the mob of fans my Mr. America win had created overseas. In fact, I ended up checking into two hotels while in London, as I was unable to stay in the first one I had booked because word had gotten out to the fans that I was staying there and they were constantly pounding on my door. I finally checked into a second hotel under an assumed name to get some peace and quiet, and to focus on the battle that I knew was ahead of me.

When the three finalists names were called out, I found myself between Drapp and Grimek. We all wanted that title, and we were all in good shape. In the judges' eyes, Grimek and I were in too good a shape, as they quickly declared the contest "a draw." We were dead even after the final round and so, to break the tie, the judging panel evoked that little line about "physical powers," a line that was open to interpretation as the sponsors and judges saw fit. One of the judges (it's been suggested that it might have been Bob Hoffman, who was Grimek's employer), suggested that the best way to break the tie was to have the stalemated pair engage in a gymnastics competition and that the Mr. Universe title would then be awarded to the better gymnast.

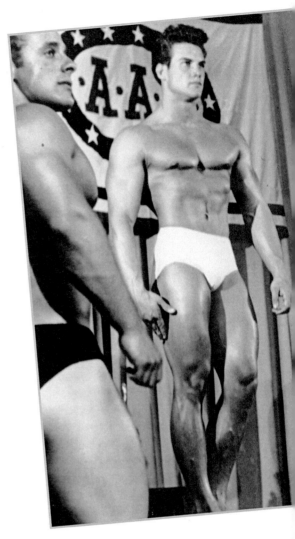

I knew right then and there that I'd lost the title. Although I could perform handstands and the like, Grimek was a gymnast par excellence. He was also an exceptional poser, having a special posing room constructed in his house that was lined with mirrors where he could spend hours perfecting his routine (which, by the way, was a joy to watch). I had entered the contest thinking that I only had to outdo Grimek in bodybuilding to win, as after all, the Mr. Universe is a physique contest. It didn't work out that way. I performed a rather shakey handstand, while Grimek did a press to handstand and then walked over into a full splits — and hit a pose. The audience went wild and John Grimek was awarded the title of Mr. Universe for 1948.

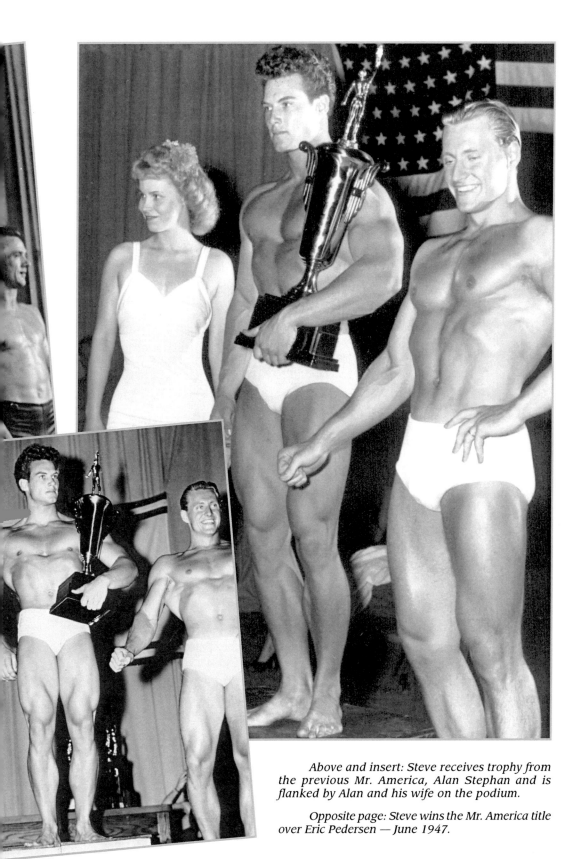

Above and insert: Steve receives trophy from the previous Mr. America, Alan Stephan and is flanked by Alan and his wife on the podium.

Opposite page: Steve wins the Mr. America title over Eric Pedersen — June 1947.

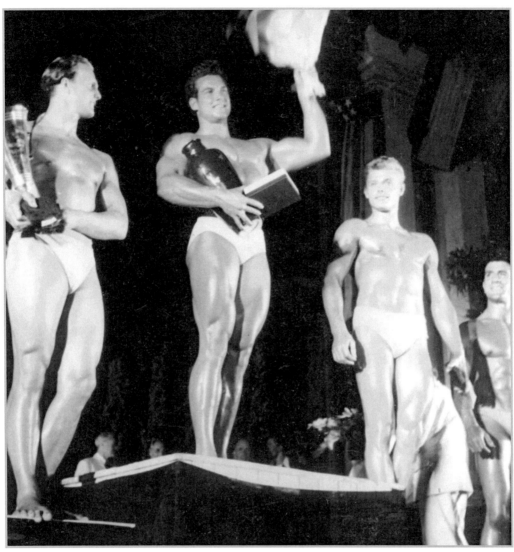
Steve accepts the laurels as Mr. World in Cannes, France — August 1948.

I shook John's hand and, as I was leaving the stage, I was approached by Oscar Heidenstam who told me that, if I could remain in Europe for another three days, there was going to be a Mr. World competition in Cannes, France on August 26, and that I would be a sure thing to win it. As I had already traveled so far, and since I definitely didn't want to return home empty handed, I decided that some time in France might be worthwhile. I easily won the contest and they also declared me "Le Plus Bel Athlete du Monde," which further served to prove to me that I had, indeed, fulfilled my ambition of improving with each outing. The Mr. America title was generally considered the "Big One," but the Mr. Universe contest, then newly created, was, by virtue of the talent it was attracting, rapidly becoming the "Super Bowl" of physique contests. And while I wanted to win the Mr. Universe, I also had to earn a living.

Upon returning to the United States, I turned my efforts towards a career in show business. Unfortunately, while my muscles were an asset in winning physique contests, they proved an absolute liability in obtaining roles in Hollywood. As most of the actors in

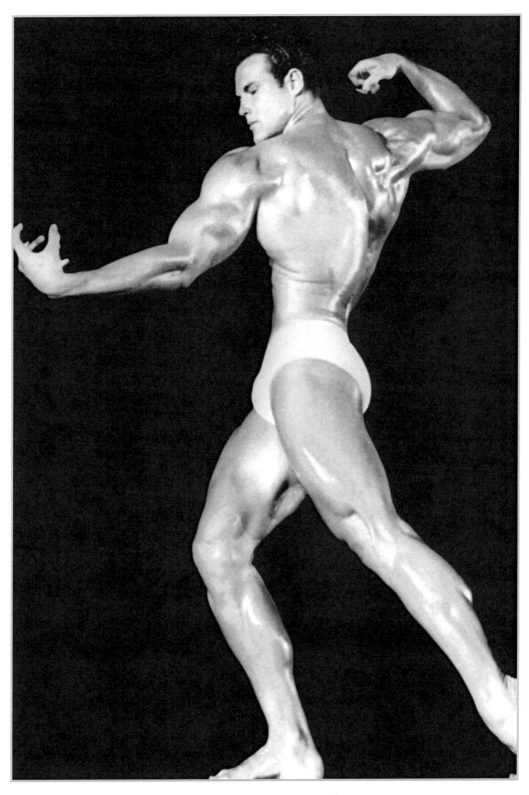

While already in Europe for London's Mr. Universe, Steve headed for France and the Mr. World contest. Above, Steve gives one of his award winning poses as he competes for the title.

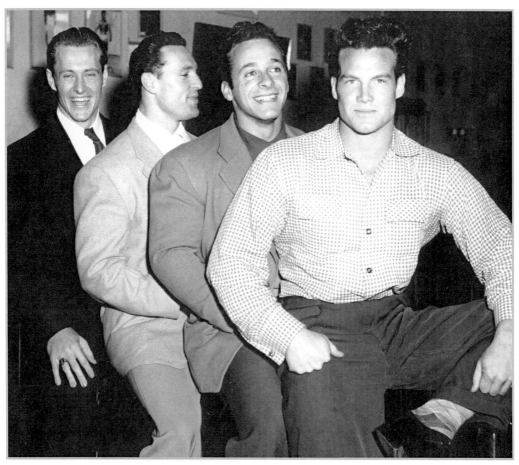

Above: A lineup of Mr. Americas — Alan Stephan (1946), Clancy Ross (1945), George Efferman (1948) and Steve Reeves (1947).

Opposite page: One of several great Mr. America publicity photos taken by Tony Lanza at Foster Avenue Beach along Chicago's lake front.

Hollywood were not physical culturists, very few of them had well-developed physiques, which made most of them insecure with my appearing alongside them. It's ironic that I would eventually be able to make my own mark in Hollywood solely because I refused to play the emaciated leading man, preferring to show audiences the beauty and value of a fully-developed male physique in films like Hercules, Duel of the Titans and The Last Days of Pompei. But back when I first began my show business career, I thought it a wiser course to do what I was told, rather than what I felt to be correct.

Once my bodyweight dropped, I appeared in the musical Kismet, guested on the Red Skelton and Dinah Shore television shows, played Li'l Abner (even at a reduced weight I always retained some degree of muscle size) and did a series of skits in some popular television and stage shows, all the while patiently awaiting my "big break." My big break, however, proved to be a long time coming, and my interests returned to my passion — bodybuilding.

In the almost two years that I'd actively been pursuing jobs in Tinsel Town, I'd hardly visited a gym. I'd lost weight on the advice of producers in order to procure film work, but I wasn't happy being a smaller me. I decided that I would take one more kick at the Mr. Universe can.

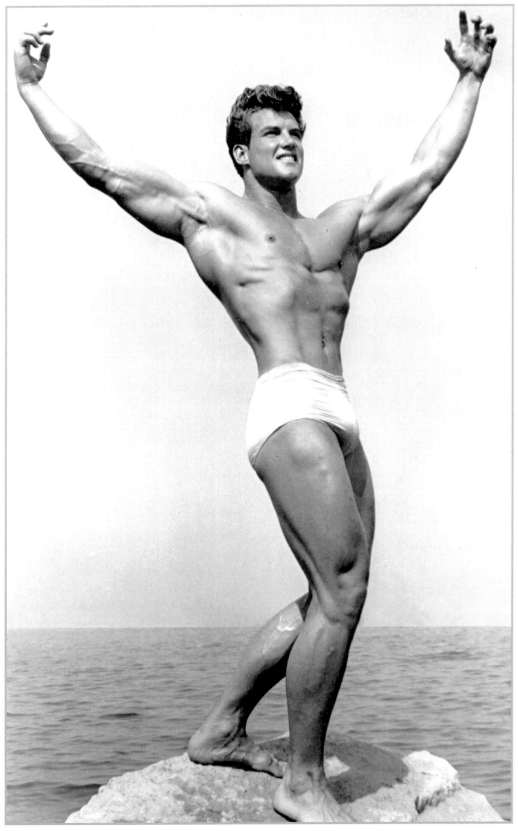

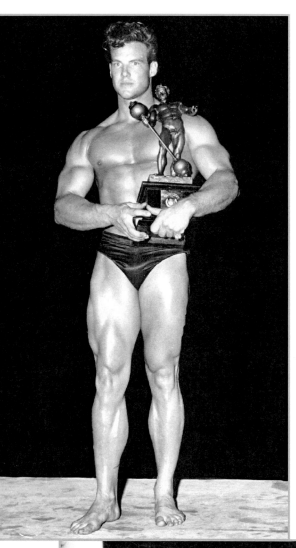

The 1950 Mr. Universe was again being held in London, England and, as it was the only title in all of bodybuilding at that time that had eluded me, I thought I'd better see if I could nail it down before walking away from the sport. There was only one problem — when I finally made up my mind to enter the contest, it was just four weeks away!

As one of my training partners, George Eiferman, was living in Pennsylvania at the time, I decided to move out East to train for the contest. I knew that my partner would push me hard, which was what I would need if I was going to be able to get into top shape in such a short time. I trained hard utilizing my Classic Physique schedule but caught pneumonia halfway through my training. That temporarily weakened and demoralized me somewhat — but surprisingly, it also served to increase my muscular definition!

Steve not only captured the Mr. Universe title, but captured the coveted Sandow statue trophy that Smythe gave to the organizers in assurance that a Britisher would win. But Mr. Universe 1950 was Steve Reeves and the treasured statue was (and still is) all his!

Class 1 Division competitors (from left to right) were Hubert Thomas of Wales, Steve Reeves of the United States of America, Reg Park of Britain and Dardenne of Belgium.

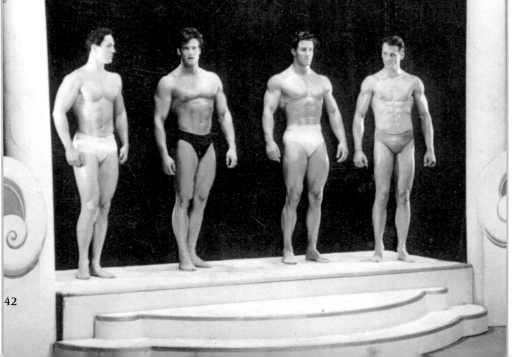

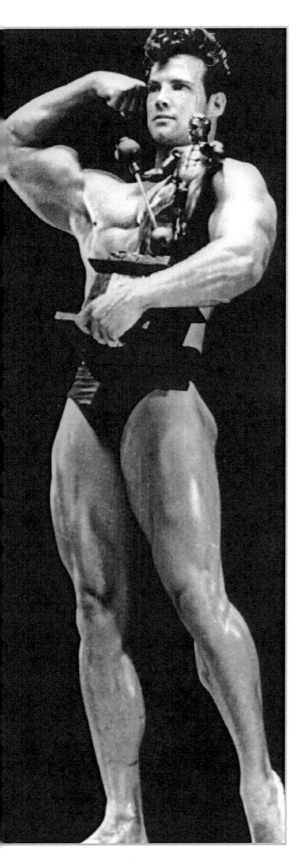

The training proved to be a tonic for me; I quickly regained muscular bodyweight, my eyes sparkled with enthusiasm, and once more I took on the look of the real Steve Reeves. Witnesses were amazed at my physical transformation and even John Grimek, whose eyes had seen everything in this sport, told me: "I can't believe it! If I hadn't seen it, I wouldn't have believed that you could have transformed your body like that in such a short span of time!" I took that as a compliment and once again boarded a plane to England.

The date of the 1950 Mr. Universe Contest was July 24, and the venue was London's Scala Theatre. My chief competition that day was a young man by the name of Reg Park, who appeared to me to be in excellent shape. The judges, however, voted in my favor and, upon winning the Mr. Universe title, I realized that this was the end of my competitive career in bodybuilding. I'd gone as high as I could go. I announced my retirement from bodybuilding competition that evening in order to refocus my attention making a go of it in movies. Yes, I was fortunate in this respect, as I made many films that were very successful on an international level. But my true passion has always been bodybuilding and trailing to build a classic physique.

In looking back over my competitive career, I realize with some measure of contentment that I accomplished what I set out to do—well, nearly everything. I always wanted to achieve a 24-inch difference between my chest and waist measurements, but I fell short of that mark by just one inch. I also wanted a shoulder breadth of 24 inches. Armand Tanny once measured me at 23-1/2. If I been able to train for six more months I'd have gotten that extra half-inch. Other than these two "failed" goals, however, I have absolutely no regrets.

What I do have, however, are loads of training secrets and numerous original bodybuilding ideas that helped me to make some of the fastest muscle gains ever recorded. And what I'd like to do in the following chapters of this book is to share them with you.

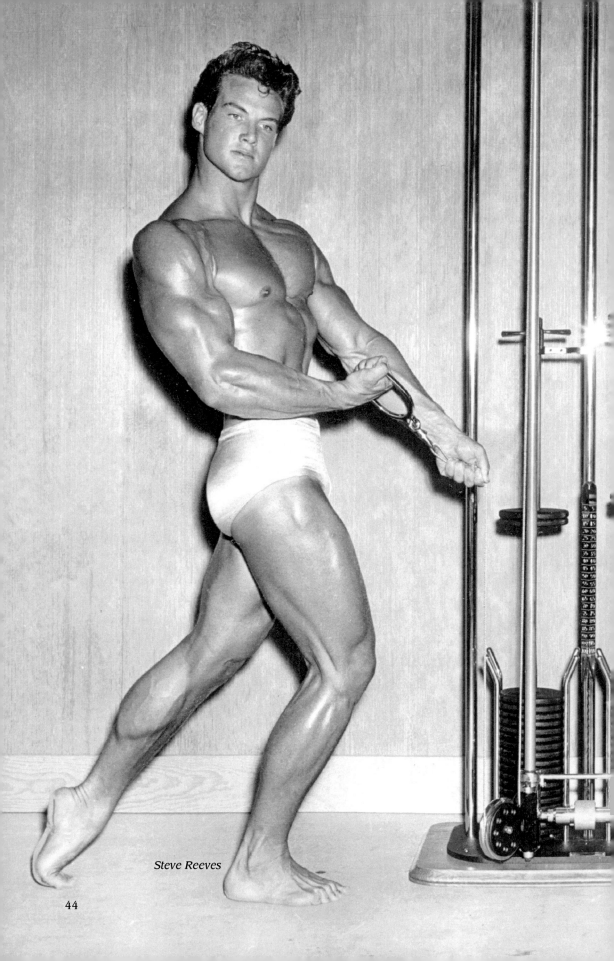
Steve Reeves

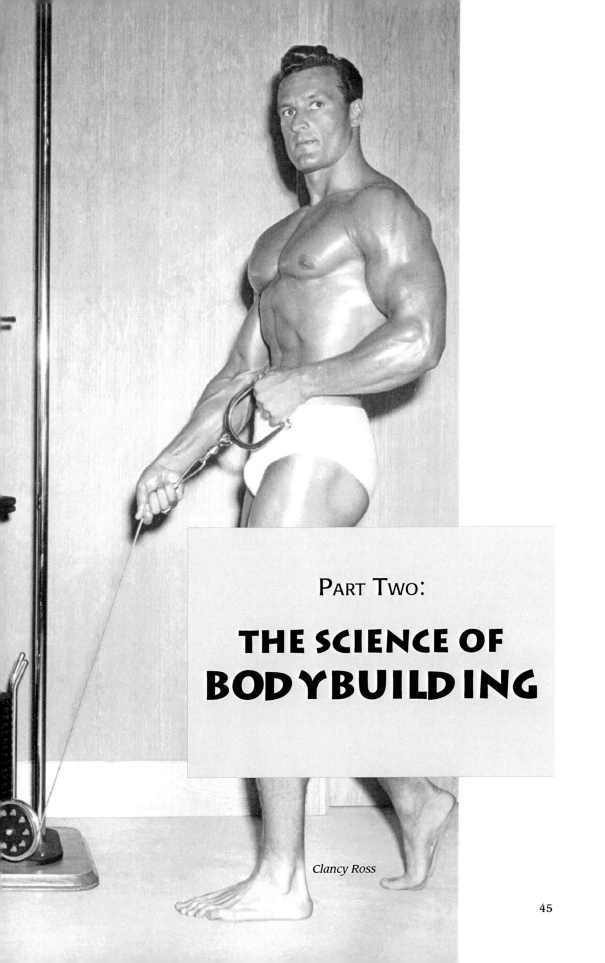

Part Two:
THE SCIENCE OF BODYBUILDING

Clancy Ross

Chapter 8: Preliminary Considerations

Before you can begin on a journey of any kind, you must first understand the terrain. Bodybuilding is no different in that it represents a journey of self-discovery; enabling you to learn the limitations and capabilities of your own body — and, believe me, no two bodies are exactly the same. With this in mind, let us examine some of the more fundamental aspects of training, the preliminary considerations, if you will.

Frequency of Training

The age-old question is just how much should you train in order to get excellent results. Are you ready? Three days a week. Does that surprise you? Well, I've never trained more than three days per week and look what it did for me!

Think about it: Training six days per week will not double your strength or size. Your muscles need rest as well as exercise. Weight training more than three days a week is overtraining! Your muscle tissue is broken down as you exercise and is rebuilding when you are at rest. Actually, most bodybuilders are overtrained and those that have done it for long periods of time are losing muscle. Since training more than three days a week is overtraining, schedule rest days in-between your training days.

Your Weekly Training Schedule

An ideal training schedule is training on Monday, Wednesday and Friday. Your rest days would be Tuesday, Thursday, Saturday and Sunday. Or, you can train Tuesday, Thursday and Saturday with rest days on Monday, Wednesday, Friday and Sunday.

The Importance of Breathing

While most of us have no trouble breathing, very few of us take the time to breathe deeply during the course of our day — and we really should. The reason being that it is oxygen that truly powers our engines (in the form of our bodies) throughout the course of a day. It is, after all, through the blood that oxygen is transported to the more than 75 trillion cells throughout our bodies. The average adult body contains about five quarts of blood traveling 1,000 separate routes. The heart muscle pumps between 5,000 and 6,000 quarts of blood daily. This blood unceasingly makes round trips throughout the body, circulating roughly once per minute when we are still, and five to six times per minute when we are active. Do you now see the need to breathe deeply? As the blood courses through our bodies, it not only takes in oxygen but picks up consumed air (carbon dioxide) for elimination through the lungs, pores, kidneys and colon.

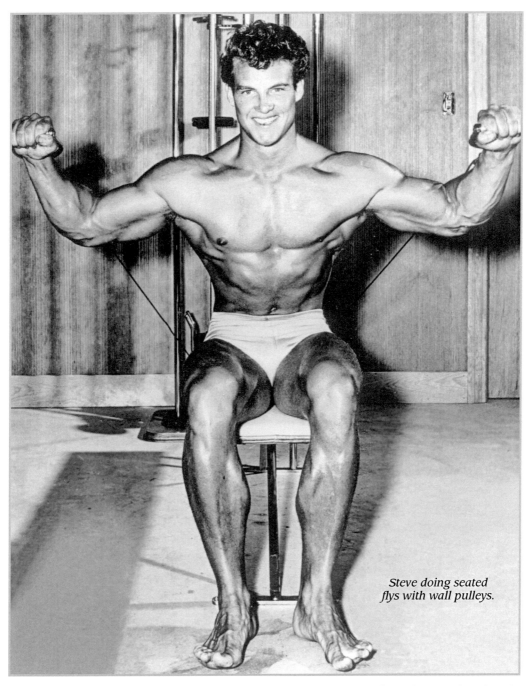

Steve doing seated flys with wall pulleys.

The blood needs to reach every little out-of-the way capillary from the top of our heads to the tips of our toes. Deep breathing should begin the first thing in the morning. In our sleep, body functions slow down and our blood pressure falls. We breathe shallowly and so there is less energy-giving oxygen in our systems when we wake up (which, incidentally, is why we typically yawn in the morning, as yawning draws more oxygen into our system). However, it is only through physical exertion that more than 10 times as much oxygen can be brought in through the lungs. A person's health and performance capacity depend predominantly on him going considerably beyond the normal resting figures for respiration, thereby increasing oxygen-supplying capacity.

Oxygen uptake of a quarter-liter per minute at rest can be increased in a trained person to five liters, or 20 times the resting value. But it's generally sufficient to frequently practice tenfold oxygen supply and for long periods of time. Power walking is perfect in this regard.

Incidentally, here's a bit of news that might well entice you to continue on with your Power Walking or oxygen uptake training. It involves a hormone called epinephrine, which is secreted by the adrenal gland. The more deeply you breathe, the more oxygen you deliver to the bloodstream, and the greater the amount of epinephrine that's processed and poured into your system. This hormone is a natural "upper" that makes you feel more alive and energetic. Deep breathing results in feeling really good without the use of pills, alcohol and tobacco. I've always felt that any unnecessary chemical taken into the body which in any way alters our delicately balanced body chemistry is an insult and a potential danger to our health, longevity and appearance.

The Value of Stretching

There are two different types of stretching: ballistic and static. Here's an overview of each.

BALLISTIC — Movements in which one group of muscles is being stretched in a bouncing and jerking manner.

STATIC — This involves holding specific joints in a locked position (only those joints that are needed) while you stretch the involved muscles and connective tissue. You then hold that stretched position for a minimum of one minute.

Both ballistic and static stretches are effective in improving flexibility. With static stretching, injuries are less likely to occur, simply because you are not exceeding the limits of the tissues being stretched. A person's inability to increase his or her range of motion can result in stretched ligaments, muscle pulls and the like. Although an increase in flexibility may decrease the chance of these injuries, too much flexibility has the potential to make joints unstable, leaving the joints vulnerable to injury.

Two more rules of safe stretching: Never stretch a cold muscle, and never stretch to the point of pain — the tightness may be uncomfortable, but if a stretch really hurts, don't go so far. A final word of advice — be careful not to overdo the stretching exercises. Always keep in mind that your goal is to increase range of motion without removing or overriding the natural safeguards built into all muscles, joints and connective tissue.

My Favorite Stretching Exercises

Straddle Stretch

The Straddle Stretch is a great flexibility movement for limbering up the lower back and hamstrings. Standing erect, I fold my arms into my chest and then bend over — making sure to keep my legs perfectly straight — until my torso is at a 90-degree angle to my legs. Once I've hit 90 degrees, I hold this position for 15 seconds. Then, I lower myself a little farther and hold this position for an additional 15 seconds. Then I lower myself still farther and again sustain this position for another 15 seconds. I lower myself once again and hold the position for a final 15 seconds, and then slowly return to the starting position. This is a great movement that I still perform today. I perform it just before going to bed, as it helps to relieve the day's tensions and also helps to keep me fluid and limber.

The Kneeling Quadriceps Stretch

This is a wonderful movement for the quadriceps muscles on the front of your thighs. To perform it, kneel on the floor with your hands on your hips. From this position, slowly draw your arms behind your torso until they are just beyond your ankles and are serving to support your torso. Now slowly lean backwards, slowly lowering yourself down towards the floor. You should feel a gentle stretch in your thighs and, once you've experienced this mild stretch, sustain this position for 60 seconds.

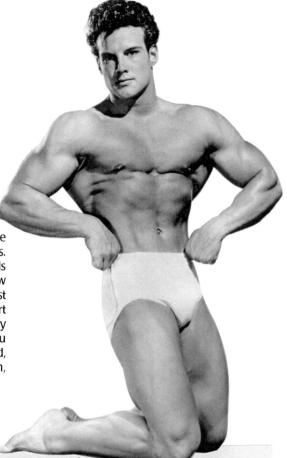

The Lunge Stretch

This works wonders for limbering up the groin or inner-thigh muscles. Start from a lunge position with your left knee forward, with hands on each side, touching the floor to help you maintain your balance. Hold this position for 30 seconds while steadily lowering your body downward to get a full stretch of your inner-thigh muscles. Then reverse your leg position and repeat the exercise for 30 seconds.

Latissimus Stretch

Latissimus stretches are a great limbering movement for the latissimus dorsi muscles of your upper back. Locate a pole or some other upright that you can grab onto that has some degree of stability. With both hands holding on to the support, place your feet up close to the support. Now, sinking your hips down and away from the support, hang on tightly with your hands, making it a point to really stretch your lats. Go down as slow as you can, making sure to keep the tension on your lats for the entire duration of the stretch (60 seconds).

Pec Stretches

To perform these properly, you'll need to stand in a doorway or between two vertical uprights, such as pillars that are close together. Placing a hand on either upright, slowly lean forward until you experience a mild stretching sensation in your pectorals or "chest" muscles. Lean forward just a little farther and sustain this stretch for 60 seconds.

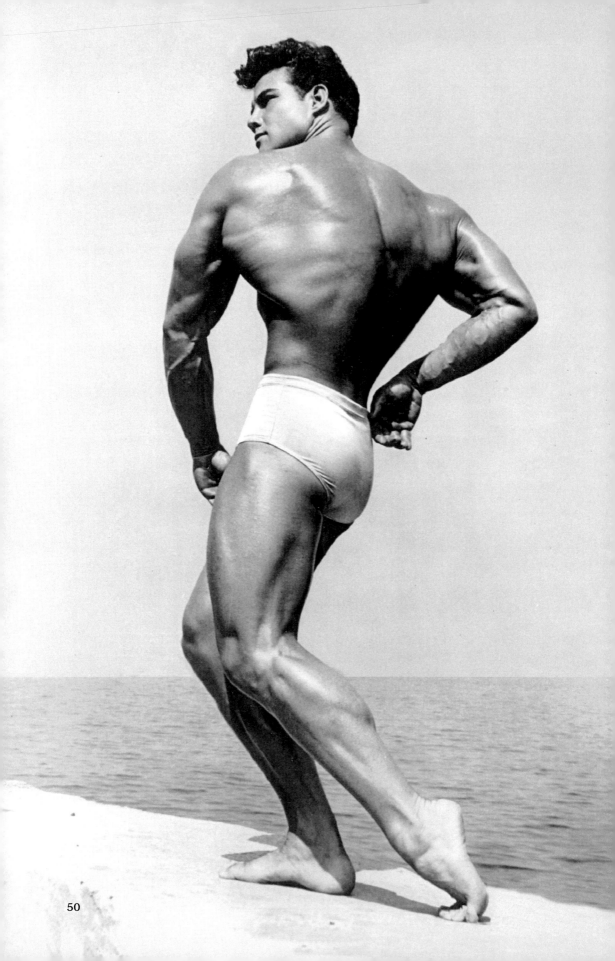

Chapter 9: No Brain, No Gain

I feel that the often used saying, "No pain, no gain" is a negative slogan and should be replaced by a more positive approach of "No brain, no gain." Be a thinking bodybuilder.

The Power of Concentration

If you really want to experience the greatest benefits from your training, you must enter a stage of deep concentration. Do not let your concentration be broken by anyone or anything. Besides, you want the time you spend in the gym to give you an hour's worth of benefit for each hour spent training.

To accomplish this, you don't have to be rude to the other members of the gym. You just politely let them know that it is your policy to practice deep concentration during your workouts and that you don't want to be disturbed during this time. Let them know that you will be happy to answer their questions and socialize before and after your workout.

When you work out using this technique of deep concentration, concentrate on doing each movement slowly through a full range of motion. Your total concentration should be only on the muscle fibers being worked. Concentrate as much on the lowering phase (the negative) of the exercise as you would on the pressing and curling (the positive).

Do not be concerned about how much weight you are using. Your purpose for coming to the gym is to develop muscle and strength—not display them! Naturally, you should use as much weight as possible while always doing the exercise in good form. Cheat only on the last rep, when your muscles are temporarily exhausted and are no longer able to do another rep in good style.

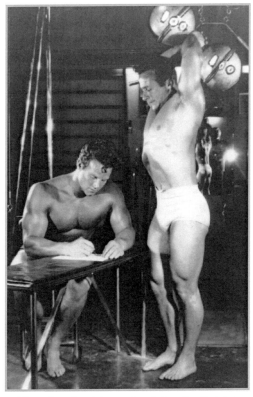
Steve logging his workout despite George Eiferman's menacing pose.

If You Can't Conceive It, You Most Likely Won't Achieve It

I want you to create a picture in your mind of how you want your physique to look when you reach your genetic potential. Then, I want you to train to achieve that image. Don't put an unachievable or unbelievable image in your mind. Don't picture yourself having the classic form of a Chris Dickerson or Frank Zane if, by nature, you are destined to have a massive musculature of a Casey Viator, Lee Haney or vice versa.

In order for you to form your overall image, you may have to draw on body parts from several different physique stars or role models for inspiration. But always keep in mind that ultimately, you must be your own body architect, your own exterior decorator.

Get in touch with your subconscious mind (the true powerhouse of your mind) by giving it positive autosuggestions. Repeat over and over that you do have the body you want and you have it right now! Affirm to yourself that you're getting stronger and more muscular every day. Repeat the words: "I think like a champion. I act like a champion. I will be a champion!"

Using these powerful affirmations will change your life very quickly. Use autosuggestion and let your subconscious mind help you create the images you consciously desire.

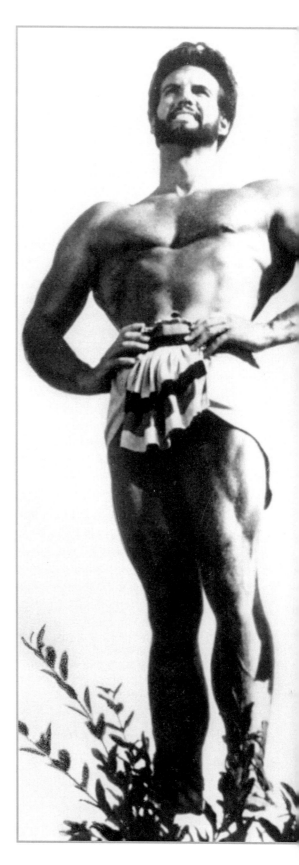

In the movie "Hercules," Steve was honored in the first Olympiad but, setting the story aside, he truly did appear to be a god among mortal men.

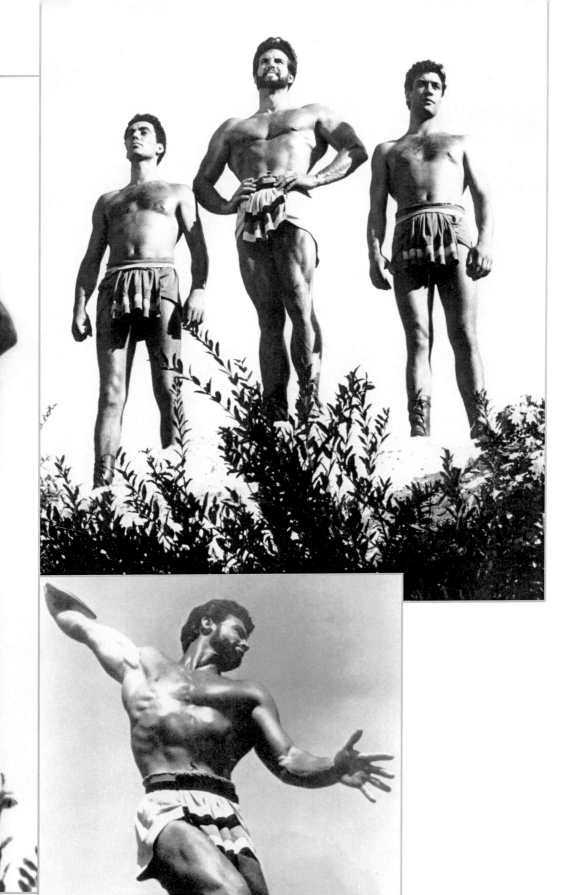

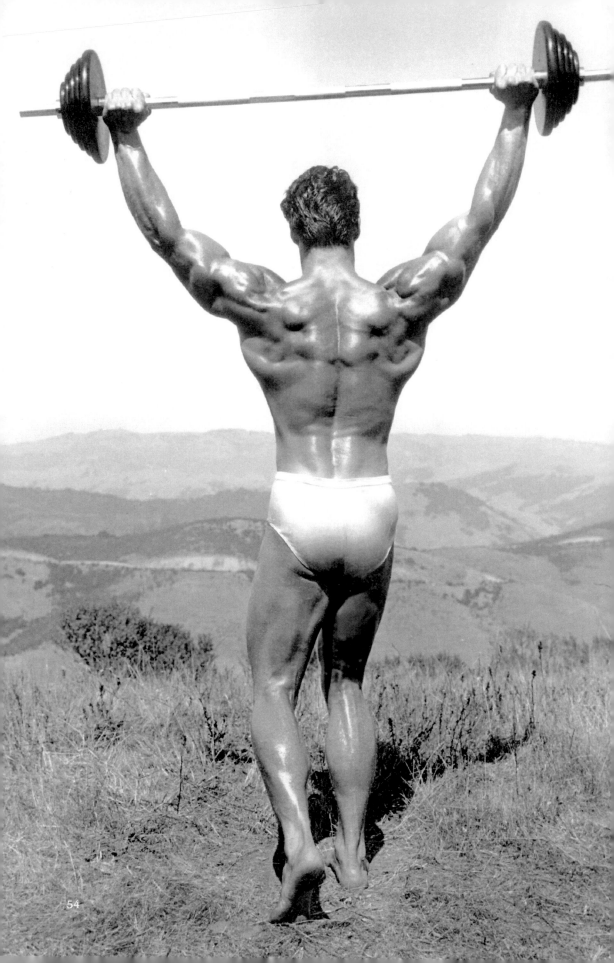

Chapter 10: Training Logic

What I'm about to tell you may shock you. That's because you've probably been so used to training a certain way for so long. Yet, I'm willing to bet that you have gotten only a fraction of the results you could be getting if you trained your body in the correct sequence. Let's look at how most bodybuilders think they should train.

Who Told You This Is the Best Way to Train?

Many people start their training by working the legs (thighs) first. The theory being that larger muscles should be worked first because they take more energy to work them than smaller muscles. Besides, if a bodybuilder would work the smaller muscles first, he wouldn't have enough energy to work the bigger muscles later in the workout. I don't agree. On the contrary, I believe that the legs should be worked near the end of your workout, after you have worked the major muscles of the upper body. Here's why:

Because the legs are the largest and strongest muscles in the body, they are needed to form a strong foundation or support while you are doing most of the exercises for the upper body. Without this strong foundation, you won't be able to put out the maximum effort while working the smaller muscles of the upper body.

I also believe it is better for your body to warm up and increase the circulation gradually by doing exercises that don't put too much demand on your system too quickly. By working the smaller muscles first, then working the legs near the end of your training, you accomplish this.

Approximately 80 percent of your blood is located in your legs and glutes (which are worked while you exercise the other body areas). So, if you work your legs first, you will be bringing even more blood down into the lower extremities, thus drawing it away from the smaller muscles in your upper body.

All of this makes for an unnecessary and undesirable demand on your system (forcing the body to pump large amounts of blood against gravity) once you start making the body bring the blood back to the upper body when you begin working the smaller muscles. The bottom line is: If you want the best results from your workouts, start with the smaller muscles of your upper body and work down to your legs.

Experience Is the Best Teacher

In working the upper body, I have found from training and observing others, that it is best to start with the deltoids. For the majority of people, the deltoids are one of the hardest muscles to completely develop. Sure, you may see some bodybuilders with a fully-developed front or side deltoid head. Yet, those bodybuilders who have all three deltoid heads (front, side and rear) fully developed, are rare indeed.

Big, wide deltoids are the mark of a great physique. They exude power and command respect. If you have fully developed shoulders, a tight midsection that displays abs, and have good calves, I guarantee you are going to have a physique that will turn heads! I strongly recommend that you work your deltoids first in your workout, when your energy level, concentration and enthusiasm are at their highest.

First the Deltoids — Then the Chest

After the deltoids are thoroughly worked and well-pumped with blood, rest for two minutes then work the chest. After hitting the chest, rest two minutes and move to the lats (upper back). This sequence allows the blood to flow with gravity downward and backward. After you've finished working the lats, take a two-minute rest.

After lats you should work the biceps (located on the front of the upper arm), and for two very good reasons. First, if you were to work your triceps (located on the back of the upper arm) before biceps, the skin on your upper arm would be so tight that you would find it difficult to get a full peak contraction while doing curls.

The other reason you want to work the biceps first is simply because they are thoroughly warmed from your just completed lat work. Movements like chins or pulldowns behind-the-neck and rows directly involve the biceps. Enough said. Work your biceps first, then take a two-minute rest before doing triceps.

After a good pump, rest two minutes and then get ready to work your quadriceps (or front thigh muscles). After hitting the quadriceps, rest two minutes and then work the hamstrings (or the back of the thigh muscles). The only time you should work your hamstrings before your quadriceps is when you're using the leg extension and leg curl machines. If you're doing squats for leg work, do the leg curls afterwards. Otherwise, if you work your quadriceps first, you won't be able to do the squats as well or use as much weight. Rest two minutes then work your calves. Rest two minutes then train your lower back. Rest two minutes then train your abs (midsection). Rest for another two minutes then work your neck.

By working your back, abs and then the neck, you're gradually bringing the blood back up from the legs and into the upper body region.

When I tell you to rest two minutes between exercises, I don't mean for you to plop yourself down on a bench and do nothing! I want you to remain standing and not sitting down. If you're not helping your training partner with a spot, keep your body in motion by walking slowly or shifting your weight from foot to foot.

For review, after a thorough warm-up, here's the order that I want you to train your body:

1) **Deltoids**
2) **Pectorals (chest)**
3) **Lats (mid and upper back)**
4) **Biceps**
5) **Triceps**
6) **Quadriceps (front thighs)**
7) **Hamstrings (back of legs)**
8) **Calves**
9) **Lower Back**
10) **Abdominals (midsection)**
11) **Neck**

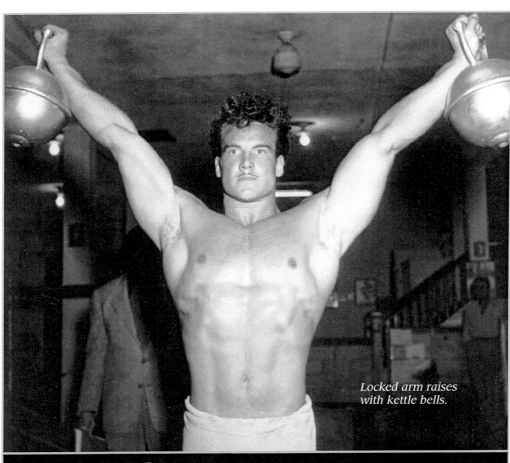
Locked arm raises with kettle bells.

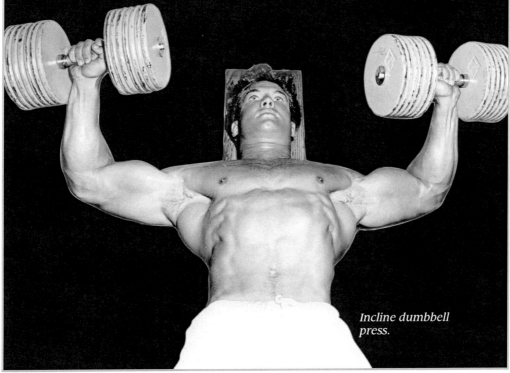
Incline dumbbell press.

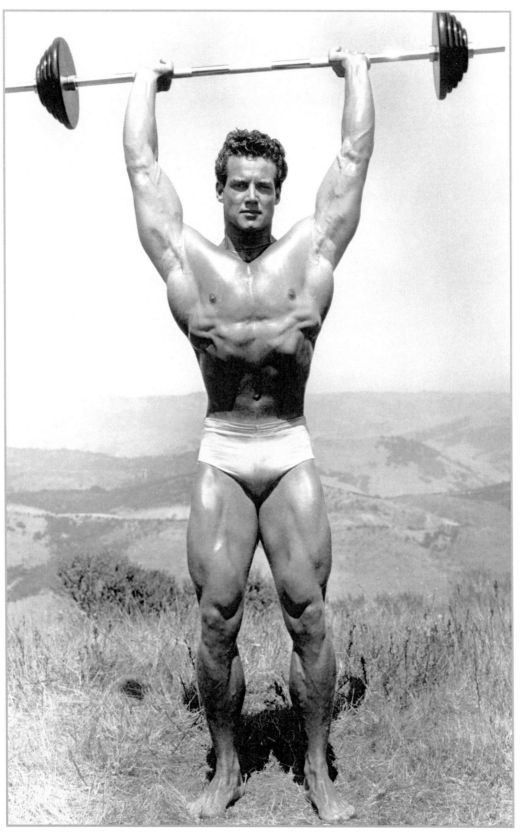

Chapter 11: High-Intensity Training

So many people, including bodybuilders and other weight-trained athletes, just don't know how to train to get the most benefit out of the time invested in their workouts. Their training program, instead of being well thought out, is haphazard at best. If you ask them why they work a certain body part first or do a certain exercise before another in their routine, they either have an illogical answer or no answer at all.

For example, they may have just seen a guy with huge arms do a set of concentration curls, so they do a set of concentration curls believing that they will get the same results. What they don't realize is that "Mr. B," with those big, well-shaped biceps, has done many basic exercises to build the foundation for those high-peaked biceps. And that concentration curls are just "putting the frosting on the cake."

If, by a rare streak of luck, they're given a logical, well thought-out routine, nine chances out of ten, they will not follow it. They'll either train too heavy or too light. Those who train too light and stop at 10 reps — because they are conditioned that 10 reps is the finish of a normal set — are just going through the motions of working out and accomplishing little else.

When their progress is not as fast as expected on their two hour per day training program, three day a week workout, they double the workout to four hours per day. They succumb to the erroneous thinking that "twice the training will yield twice the results twice as fast." The reality is that twice 25 percent intensity is only 50 percent intensity — not nearly enough for truly spectacular results.

On the other side of the coin are those that use weights that are too heavy to lift with strict style. They swing, they bounce, they bend under or cheat any way they can just to finish their set. They should concentrate on developing their strength and not demonstrating it. Strength demonstrations should be performed only at contests and shows and not in the training room. A truly strong person can impress and inspire thousands from the stage. Who are you impressing in the gym? A few newcomers? The guys that have been working out for a while are more concerned about what they're doing and not how much weight you are using.

In order to get the most benefit from your workouts in the shortest time, you must choose the right system of training for your specific goal. If your main goal is strength, you will work out doing near-maximum lifts; low reps of two and three for five to six sets, with rest periods of up to five minutes between sets.

If you want a combination of strength and muscular growth, you should use near maximum weights. Perform moderately low reps of five to six for five to six sets, with rest periods of two to three minutes in between sets.

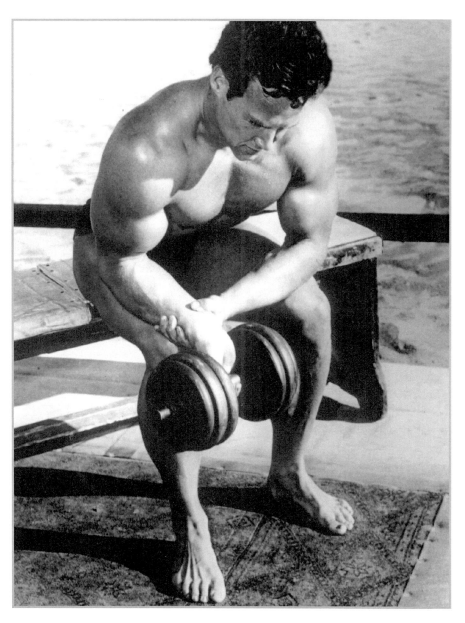

Above: Steve shows how a properly done wrist curl affects the biceps.

Right: The two photos demonstrate calf raises at different intensities in training.

For maximum muscular development, use the maximum weight you are able to do in good form for 8 to 12 reps. By good form I mean doing each rep slowly and smoothly — without swinging or bouncing to create momentum or centrifugal force — on the way up and down. Each rep should take you approximately two seconds to do the positive portion of the movement and three seconds to do the negative or lowering part of the exercise. The degree of intensity used in a training session depends on the following eight factors:

When you are selecting a workout schedule, keep these eight factors in mind:

1) **The amount of weight used**
2) **The speed of the movement**
3) **The number of repetitions performed**
4) **The duration of pause between reps**
5) **The number of sets performed**
6) **The amount of rest between sets**
7) **The strictness of form used**
8) **The duration of the training period**

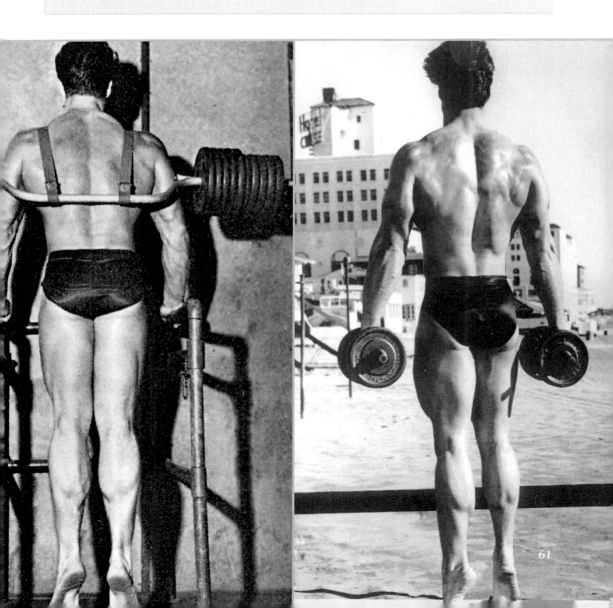

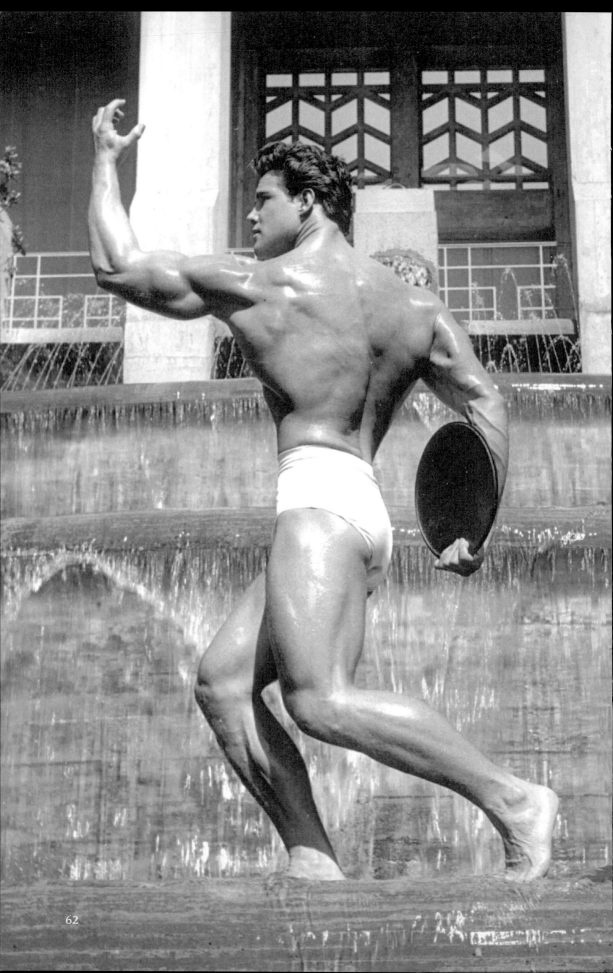

Chapter 12:
Building The Classic Physique — First Principles

For the last 20 or so years, the image of the ideal male physique has been and continues to be distorted by the bulk-crazy judges. Not only that, but all of this is perpetuated by the majority of the bodybuilding magazines for their own financial gains. Disappointingly, this is done with little, if any, regard as to what impression the bulky image they are promoting and encouraging has on the uninitiated person on the street.

Maybe you've been one of them. Well, I've got good news for you. You're learning how to make your physique a truly classic one. And a select few of the bodybuilding magazines have had the courage and concern for the sport to come out with articles and editorials against bulking up, and in favor of proportion and symmetry. They are to be commended for their efforts.

Too much size doesn't make a good impression or gain admiration and respect for the sport of bodybuilding. You may say, "Well everyone looks at a guy that is really bulked up." Yes they do, but are they looking with admiration, curiosity or thinking that he should be in a freak show? Don't forget that these same people will also gawk at a man who stands 7-feet tall and weighs 300 pounds. And who, if they had their choice, would want to be 7-feet tall unless they wanted to be a basketball star?

Yes, if there was a magic button people could press to make them 6-feet-2-inches tall, with fabulous proportion and symmetry, they wouldn't hesitate to press it. Please don't get me wrong. I'm not putting down great physiques such as Arnold Schwarzenegger and Sergio Oliva. These champions were tremendous goal-setters and through years of hard work, dedication and a bathtub full of sweat, went on to build two of the greatest physiques the sport will ever see.

As I look back on their careers and many of those who've come and gone, I just can't help but think that they could've done a much better job of promoting and popularizing weight training if only they hadn't succumbed to the muscle magazine propaganda of BIGGER IS BETTER AND BULK IS BEAUTIFUL. The bottom line is that the majority of the blame for this craziness should be placed on the physique judges who emphasized bulk, under the guise of proportion, and sorely neglected the absolute beauty of a human body that is balanced and symmetrical.

I'm going to tell it to you straight: If the judges had concentrated more on judging for proportion and symmetry, along with muscular definition and size, and judged with a uniformity of standards, the Schwarzeneggers, Olivas, Nubrets and others of that caliber would still have been great physique stars. The big difference is that the others wouldn't have had to spend so many years taking growth-enhancing substances to gain that extra bulk to become champions.

The Standards of Symmetry

We are all born with bodies that differ from one another. No two are exactly alike. So how can we set a standard for muscular size that will be fair to everyone and still be symmetrical?

We all have a bone structure that is, in most cases, in proportion to our height. A man that is 5-feet-6-inches usually doesn't wear a size 7-1/2 hat and a pair of size 12 shoes, such as a man 6-foot-4-inches would. With this is mind, I have developed the following method of predicting the potential maximum symmetrical proportions for each individual male based on height and bone size.

Classic Physique Proportions*

Arm size = 252% of wrist size

Calf size = 192% of ankle size

Neck size = 79% of head size

Chest size = 148% of pelvis size

Waist size = 86% of pelvis size

Thigh size = 175% of knee size

Weight = 295% of height

The above proportion guidelines are calculated to be the maximum measurements for a well-developed, balanced and symmetrical physique.

* Please note that this chart was calculated for men and the "percentages" will vary slightly from one man to another without changing the overall symmetry.

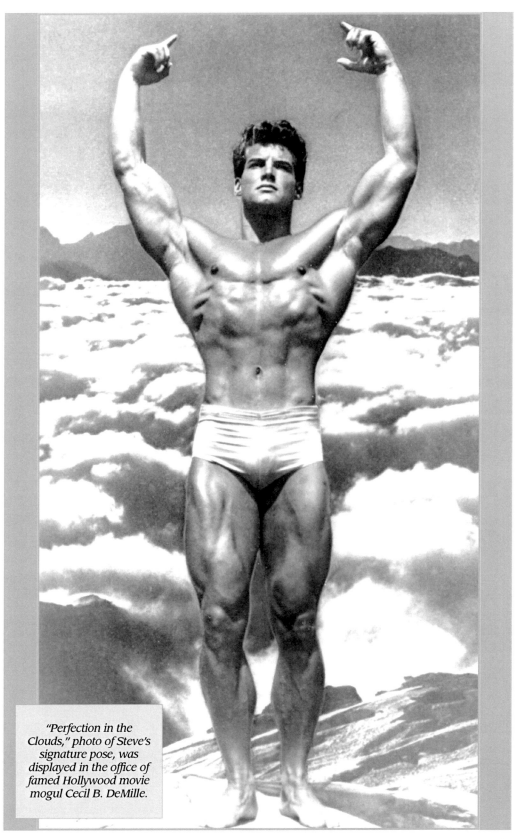

"Perfection in the Clouds," photo of Steve's signature pose, was displayed in the office of famed Hollywood movie mogul Cecil B. DeMille.

Chapter 13: What Is the "Classic Physique"?

I've spoken throughout this book about the ideal of achieving the Classic Physique, so many of you are probably wondering just what a classic physique is — which I'll be happy to explain in this chapter. A classic physique is one that is in perfect proportion — or as close as possible to it. And by proportion, I mean the calves, the neck and the biceps should measure exactly the same. Also, you should strive for wide shoulders, small waist and hips and everything else in proportion.

Avoid Trapezius and Oblique Emphasis

In building the classic physique, shy away from exercises that stress the trapezius muscle at the base of the neck, because the bigger the traps are, the narrower your shoulders appear. Instead of a square-shouldered look, a person with overdeveloped traps looks round-shouldered.

Another thing to avoid is training your oblique muscles of the midsection. If you build these muscles up too much, your waist will look wider, detracting from your broad-shouldered appearance.

I got the idea for formulating these "classic" proportions from looking at Jack LaLanne, who had a big chest and a small waist — in fact, Jack had a 20-inch difference between the measurement of his chest and waist. I always wanted to build a 24-inch differential between my waist and my chest — and that became my goal. I focused my diet and training to achieve a minuscule waist and a maximally developed chest and back. I actually built this chest/waist differential up to 23 inches but then I went into the movies and actually had to undo a lot of the muscle building I'd done, so that I didn't dwarf my fellow actors. I never reached that 24-inch differential, but having that goal in mind served to keep my training on the right track and led to me cultivating a classic physique.

Similarly, I wanted to build a shoulder span of two feet from one tip of the deltoid to the other. The closest I ever got to this goal was 23-1/2 inches — I had my good friend Armand Tanny measure me with a pair of outside calipers — but then I had to lose weight to make another film and never reached this goal either. It's ironic, but these are the only two goals I ever set for myself that I never obtained. But simply having them served to keep my training on the correct track and I never once tried to build size simply for the sake of getting "bigger." Everything has to be in proportion and geared toward creating a "classic" or pleasing, proportionate look.

The Steve Reeves' Proportion Chart

In building my own physique, and in training others to build theirs, I always emphasized the necessity of proportion and symmetry. To this end, I devised a chart of sorts that allows one to determine whether or not he is at an ideal weight for his height and thus, if he's en route to building a classic physique. Here is the chart:

Height:	Classic Physique Weight:
5' 5"	160 pounds
5' 6"	165 pounds
5' 7"	170 pounds
5' 8"	175 pounds
5' 9"	180 pounds
5' 10"	185 pounds
5' 11"	190 pounds
6'	200 pounds
6' 1"	210 pounds
6' 2"	220 pounds
6' 3"	230 pounds
6' 4"	240 pounds
6' 5"	250 pounds

The chart figures are calculated with a medium-boned man in mind. If you have heavy bones, you can add 10 pounds to the height/weight calculations chart; if you have light bones, you can subtract 10 pounds.

Our base model for these calculations stands six feet tall and weighs 200 pounds. As you can see, the formula is that for every inch a person is over six feet in height, muscle weight should increase 10 pounds. Similarly, for the first inch in height below six feet, weight should decrease 10 pounds. Below a height of 5-feet-11-inches, weight should decline five pounds for every inch of height.

These are figures that I've arrived at after training or studying the physiques of many champion athletes in many different sports. Once a person exceeds his ideal weight for his height, he becomes out of proportion and not only no longer possesses a "classic" physique, but doesn't function optimally either.

Classic Physique Training Objectives

When someone comes into a gym to build a classic physique, he/she should not be concerned with simply adding size for the sake of adding size, or in lifting heavy weights simply for the sake of lifting heavy weights. You must have a purpose or a reason for your training and that reason should be tempered with only one word — PROPORTION. You must apply training logic to your endeavors.

These tips are helpful when proportion is your goal:

Complete Extension and Complete Contraction

You must exercise your muscles through their fullest possible range of motion. This means complete extension and complete contraction in perfect style — but get every last rep you can from every set you perform.

Have a Workout Partner

Having a workout partner has several advantages. I've always found that one solid training partner was perfect because, apart from the motivation he'll give you, the timing for rest in between sets seems perfect. When he's doing his set, you're resting, and when you're doing your set, he's resting. And the rest periods — usually between 45 seconds to

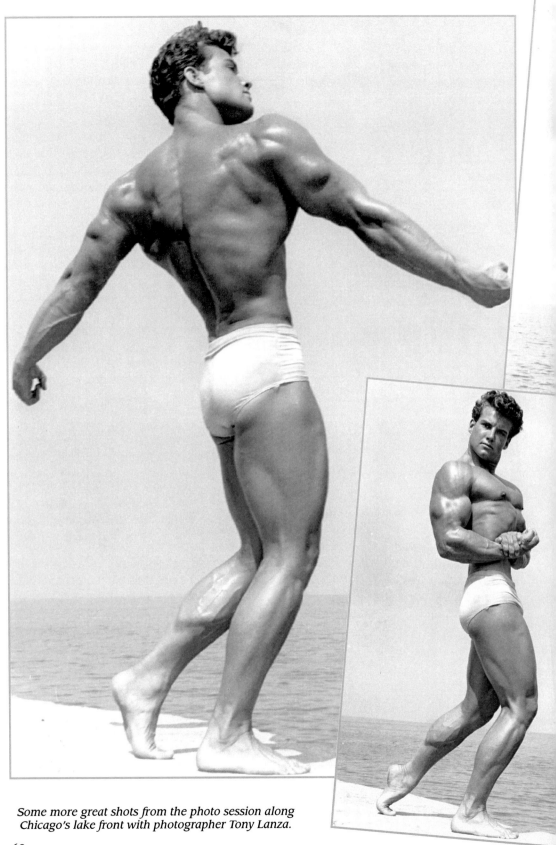

Some more great shots from the photo session along Chicago's lake front with photographer Tony Lanza.

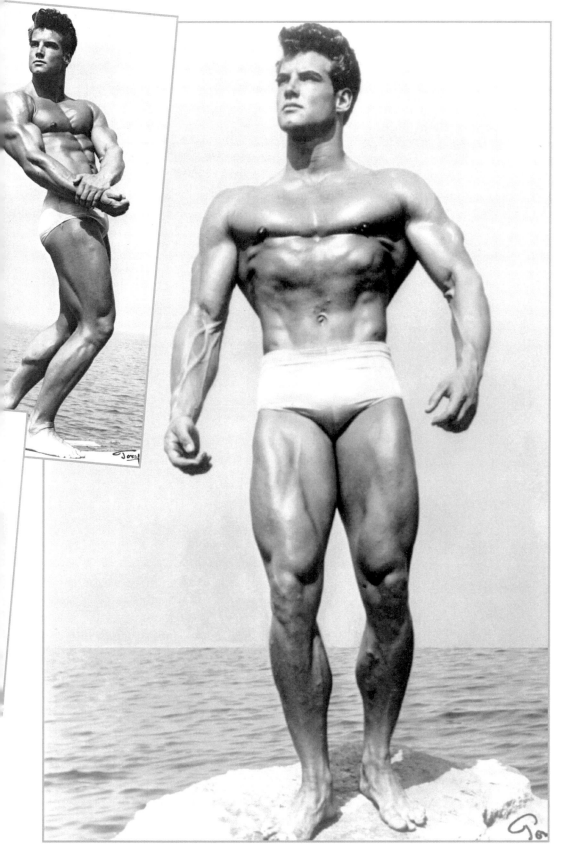

one minute in length — allow you to recover sufficiently to put your all into each and every set. I've experimented in the past with additional workout partners, such as training with two or three guys, but I've found that I cooled down too much while waiting my turn to perform a set for such a structure to be efficient or effective.

Training with only one partner keeps your enthusiasm high; when he's performing his set you can encourage him, count his reps for him (which allows him to focus more on the muscle contracting), and he does likewise for you. I've had the best and most productive workouts of my career with one reliable workout partner. And always select a partner who has the same workout goals and enthusiasm that you do — or even more, if possible!

Train Wide to be Wide

I've always believed that if you think wide and train wide, you'll become wide. That's why I do a lot of wide-grip exercises—like wide-grip bench presses, wide-grip chins behind neck, press behind neck with a wide grip, and so on.

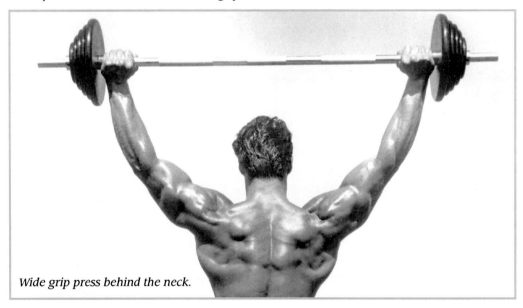
Wide grip press behind the neck.

Contrasting Ideals: The Classic vs. Contemporary Physique

The majority of physiques I see today lack the one thing that is primary to the classic physique—proportion. Easily 90 percent of the bodybuilders I see competing today lack, for example, the calf development to match their arms or neck. The trapezius muscle is always overdeveloped so that they can engage in their "crab" or "most muscular" poses, but then they suffer the narrow-shoulder syndrome when not engaged in a total flex-out.

Don't misunderstand me, the trapezius is a good muscle to develop—for supreme strength. If you're a competitive weightlifter or powerlifter, then you need that trapezius development to generate the extreme power required to make heavy lifts. But if your goal is to have a good physique, and be strong (if not necessarily the world champion in a strength sport), then you don't need that extra development in the trapezius.

Also, a lot of champion bodybuilders today lack any individuality to their physiques. They all look the same — and with good reason: they all train the same. They eat the same, perform the same routines, take the same steroids and other supplements. They are no longer individuals.

In my day, you could identify people — and bodybuilding champions to be sure — from hundreds of yards away by the specific and very distinct shape of their physiques. I could always tell Clancy Ross, Alan Stephan and John Grimek from 100 yards away. Nowadays, when viewed from a distance, all bodybuilders look the same.

Too many people today blindly follow somebody else's dictates. They'll see somebody with big arms and they'll do the routine that this individual utilizes — not that his program will necessarily work for them. Or they'll fall victim to training their strongest or best body part to bizarre and downright freakish dimensions — but at the expense of what they should be concentrating on with their training — symmetry and proportion.

Typically someone will be working out in the gym and a member will come over and say, "Hey man, what great legs you've got!" So then the guy will work his legs more and more until they get way out of proportion. Many of you reading this are probably familiar with former bodybuilding champion Tom Platz — he was a case in point of the above syndrome. At one point they complimented him so much on his legs that he trained them right out of proportion — that wasn't a classic physique at all. Fortunately, Tom stepped back and assessed the situation and began to train his upper body with the same fury for which he was renowned for training his legs. Still, the damage had been done and he was never able to successfully correct his lower-body imbalance. Admittedly, he built a rugged, Herculean physique — but not a classic one.

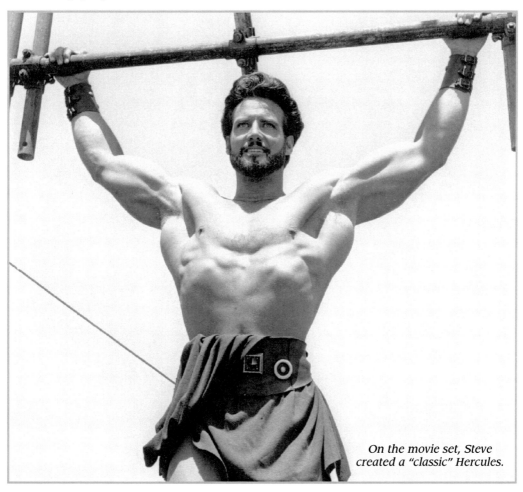

On the movie set, Steve created a "classic" Hercules.

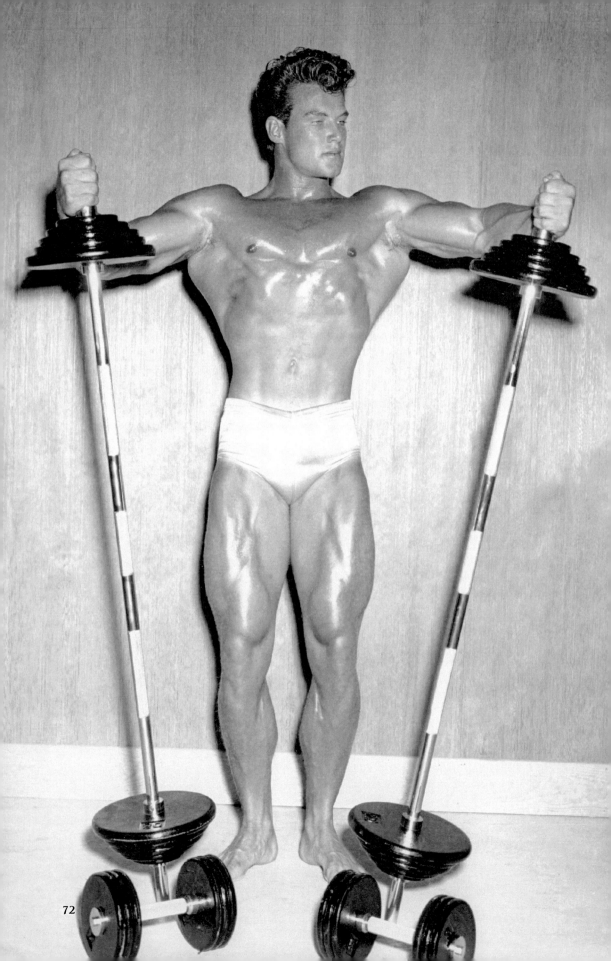

Chapter 14: Building The Classic Physique — The Routine

Now that we know what a Classic Physique is, let's get down to the business of building it. Through many years of careful thought, research and observation, I created a routine that took into account all of the necessary ingredients for building a proportionate, classic physique. I used this routine to build my body up to its all-time best shape. Best of all, it builds muscle that endures.

When I was making movies in Europe, I only had to train one month a year to tune up my muscles to look good on screen — simply because they never really went away. My shoulders were always broad, my waist always trim and my neck, arms and calves always measured the same — as a result of my having trained diligently on the routine that I'm about to relate to you in this chapter.

Acknowledge the Weights — But Follow the Schedule

What follows, then, are the exact same exercises, sets, reps and — where applicable — poundages I utilized to create my own classic physique. The weights I employed are, obviously, what my muscles allowed me to utilize with optimum efficiency, and are presented here only as a guide. Just like the height/weight chart outlined in the last chapter, your training poundages will vary according to such personal factors as your height and bone structure. However, the exercises, sets and reps I'm about to list will bring about a tremendous change in your physical appearance, and lead you well on your way to creating a classic physique of your own. Now, let's get to it!

The Warm-up

Dumbbell Swing Through

Sets: 1

Reps: 20

You should always precede your workout with a thorough warm-up. You can use a stationary bike, a treadmill or any apparatus that will serve to decrease viscosity of the joints and to elevate your pulse rate. Upon completion (five minutes or so), take hold of a dumbbell and perform 20 repetitions of dumbbell swings.

The motion consists of grasping a light dumbbell (I used to use 20 pounds) and, with your feet spread a little wider than shoulder-width apart, place the dumbbell between your legs (half squat) and as far behind you as possible. From this position, straighten and swing the dumbbell upward over your head as far as you can reach. Immediately return to the starting position and repeat for 20 repetitions. The dumbbell swing is a great total-body warm-up exercise that will really prepare your muscles for the workout to come.

The Workout: ❶ Deltoids

I always trained my shoulders first in my workouts in order to emphasize the proportion factor. I typically performed three sets of three movements, each of which was geared to target a different aspect of the deltoids. My repetitions were always between 8 and 12. This would give me nine sets per body part.

Upright Rowing (front delt emphasis)

Reps: 8-12

Sets: 3

Make it a point to "lock" your lats into place by flexing them hard throughout the movement. This will effectively disengage your trapezius muscles from kicking in and performing the majority of the work. You want to really target your front deltoids (although the side deltoids also receive tremendous stimulation from this movement) with this exercise, so focus entirely on this muscle group throughout the duration of your sets.

You will perform three sets of 8 to 12 reps here. I used to use a down-the-rack system of training with most exercises – and certainly with this one. In other words, I would start out my first set with my top weight and then reduce the weight slightly with each succeeding set.

Typically, I'd start out with 130 pounds and then I'd go to 120 pounds and finally, depending upon how I felt, I would either stay with the 120 pounds or else reduce the weight further to 110 pounds – it all depends on your power of recuperation.

The reason I always started with my top weight was that, if you're already warmed up and you give your first set your supreme effort, then there's no way you're immediately going to be able to put out the same energy for your second set (simply because you used it up in the performance of your first set) — unless you had a lot of rest, which would defeat the entire purpose.

Press-Behind-Neck
(wide-grip – side delt emphasis)

Reps: 8-12

Sets: 3

This movement can be performed either seated or standing. I usually did mine standing up. Taking hold of an Olympic bar, raise it from the floor to your shoulders in one smooth motion. From this position, press the bar smoothly overhead.

Once the bar reaches full extension, lower it back down – but this time let the bar come down BEHIND your head until it rests on your trapezius muscle at the base of your neck.

Once it rests on your traps, take a wide grip on the bar and smoothly press it back up to the fully-extended position and repeat, lowering it behind your head each time.

Bent-Over Lateral Raises
(rear delt emphasis)

Reps: 8-12

Sets: 3

This is a great exercise for the rear deltoids. Holding two moderately weighted dumbbells, bend over at the waist until your torso is at a 90-degree angle to your legs.

Keeping your arms perfectly straight, raise the dumbbells laterally out to the sides and upward until they are parallel with your shoulders then pause in the fully-contracted position for a second or so before lowering the dumbbells back down – still keeping your arms straight – in front of your thighs.

The Workout: ❷ Chest

Barbell Bench Press (wide-grip)

REPS: 8-12

SETS: 3

I would adjust my arms wide enough (almost touching the inside collars on the barbell) so that I would have a steady degree of demand placed on the muscle from beginning to end. The grip on this movement is very important because, if your grip is too close, you'll have an easy start and a difficult finish; and if your grip is too wide, you'll have a hard start and an easy finish. I found that an in-between grip that is still wide — but not too wide (you'll have to experiment for yourself to find out where this grip will be on the bar) — will result in an even amount of tension placed upon the muscles from beginning to end.

Dumbbell Incline Press
(pronating grip)

REPS: 8-12

SETS: 3

For this exercise, I would take hold of two heavy dumbbells and lie back on an incline bench that was angled at 45 degrees. I'd lower the dumbbells to my chest with my palms facing forward (my thumbs would be facing each other) and then, as I pressed the dumbbells upwards, I would turn my palms so that they were facing each other (my thumbs would then be facing the wall behind me at the completion of the movement) and touch the dumbbells at the top of the movement.

Remember: lowering — thumbs in; raising — thumbs up until you reach half way, then turn the palms in. Performing your repetitions this way will really maximize your pectoral contraction. The elbows should travel parallel to the body and you should lower the dumbbells until both the elbow and the shoulder are parallel to the floor.

Again, I'd use a down-the-rack principle, starting with 110 pounds, then 105, then 100 pound dumbbells. At Yarick's Gym, the heaviest dumbbells they had were 110 pounds, so I never trained seriously with dumbbells any heavier than that (I remember once using a pair of 115's but it didn't feel as good as the 110's).

Flying Motion (flat bench)

REPS: 8-12

SETS: 3

I'd like to stress that this movement which has come to be known today as dumbbell flyes is not a lateral movement — which is what some personal trainers preach. Again, you start the movement with your arms fully extended and in the thumbs-in position.

However, this time your thumb should be pressed against the inside of the plate with the rest of the dumbbell hanging down and resting against your forearm. This results in an offset grip on the dumbbells, which helps to keep sustained tension on your pectorals throughout the movement.

You should keep your arms slightly bent throughout the movement. When I did this movement, I used to imagine that my arm was immobilized in a plaster cast, at a slightly bent angle that would never change. Your arm should be bent at a slight angle — and you should keep it at that angle throughout the entire motion, from full extension to full contraction.

On this exercise — while I stress full extension, you have to be careful because your shoulder joint is a delicate articulation and subject to injury rather easily. With this in mind, full extension in this movement should not exceed a comfortable stretch — don't hyperextend your arms. I used to use 65-pound dumbbells with repetitions in the 8 to 12 range for three all-out sets.

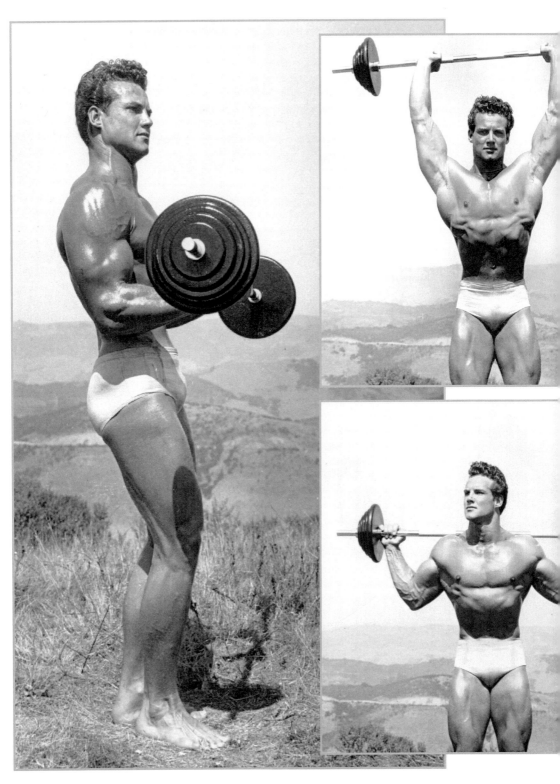

Above photo has Steve doing a standing barbell curl — with palms up grip and elbows pressed in tightly, he slowly curls the barbell up until it almost touches his chin.

Insert photos show press behind neck — he clears from floor to shoulders pressing the bar smoothly overhead, lowers it behind his neck taking a wide grip, and presses smoothly back up.

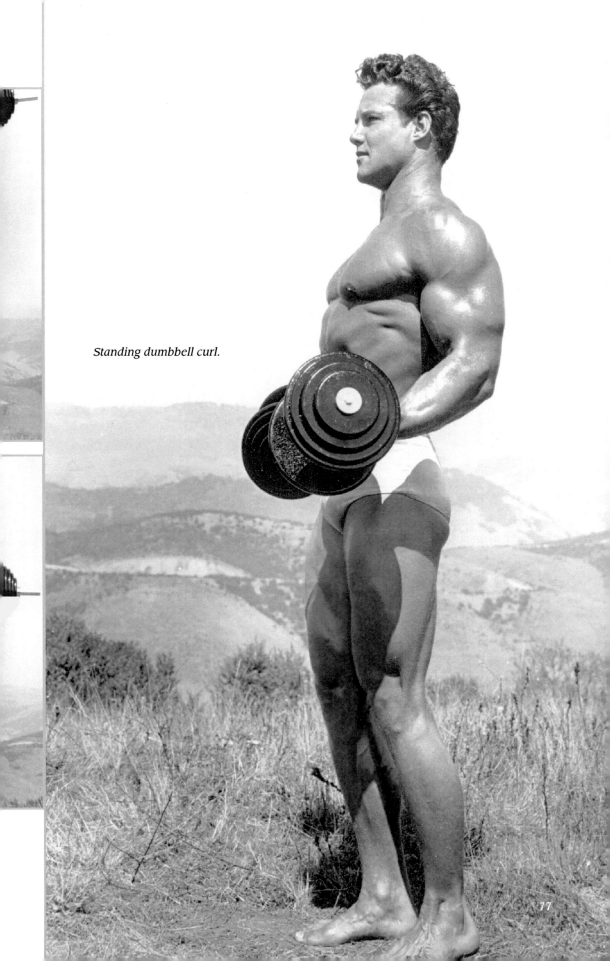

Standing dumbbell curl.

The Workout: ❸ Lats

Chin-Behind-Neck or Lat Pulldown-Behind-Neck

Reps: 8-12

Sets: 3

Start lat training with either of these exercises using a wide grip. If you have someone to hold you down (so that you can maximize the weight you use), you can do pulldowns behind the neck using an overhead pulley or "lat machine," or else do them on a chin-up bar by yourself. Either way, I would recommend no more than three sets of either exercise.

When performing chins I would sometimes add a 20-pound plate around my waist to make those reps difficult (some may only need to use a 10-pound plate — or no extra weights at all) or, if you're using the overhead pulley, put the maximum on the stack that you can use in good form and have a buddy or training partner hold you down so that you can perform the movement without also fighting to sustain your position on the floor.

Low Pulley Lat Pull
(seated cable rows)

Reps: 8-12

Sets: 3

On the low pulley lat pull you should be seated — but remember to keep your body leaning forward at all times and just bring your arms back and forth.

I notice that a lot of people, including people who have won Mr. Olympia, will grab hold of the low pulley row handle (typically a V-bar, using a palms-in grip) and just heave and jerk their whole body back and forth. They're working their whole body, but doing nothing to target the lats as well as they could if they sustained the leaning forward position and only concentrated on moving their arms.

Work your lats — not your lower back!

I believe the reason that most people torque their bodies so much is simply to use more weight and show off at the gym — but this should never be your objective if building a classic physique is your goal. They would get more benefits — that is, more results in a shorter period of time — if they simply forgot about the weight and concentrated on doing the movement correctly. Again, I used to use between 150 and 170 pounds on this movement, just focusing on a long, smooth contraction and extension.

One-Arm Row (dumbbell)

Reps: 8-12

Sets: 3

The best way to perform one-arm dumbbell rows is to take hold of a dumbbell in one hand and then lean over and place your other arm on a flat bench. Keep the leg (the one on the opposite side of the body in which you are holding the dumbbell) slightly bent and slightly in front of the other leg, which should be kept straight. Pull the dumbbell up from a position parallel to the lead foot to your hip in one smooth motion, and then lower the dumbbell under control back to the position next to your foot again.

Do not raise the dumbbell up to your chest — never lift it any higher than the hip. Again, do this exercise for three sets of 8 to 12 repetitions, doing both sides of the body each set (rather than finishing three sets for the right side, then switching hands).

I liked to utilize an 80-pound dumbbell when I was performing this movement, then stretch my lats. I'd go over to the squat rack, grab the horizontal support bar, pull back and down to stretch my lats — it always felt great after a hard lat workout to stretch them out immediately afterwards.

The Workout: ❹ Biceps

After all of the preceding lat work, your biceps are going to be thoroughly warmed up — so now is the perfect time to train them! When I first started out, I used to use three biceps exercises: barbell curls, dumbbell curls and concentration curls. However, years later I found out that incline dumbbell curls were the best possible biceps exercise. When I was in the Army I recall trying an experiment of sorts: I would see how many different exercises I could think of for each muscle group and do them one at a time — and then next day I would see what part of the muscle was sore, thereby indicating which part of the muscle the exercise was effective in training.

I only had a 100-pound set of weights, so I would think of an exercise and wait a week in order to ensure maximum recovery of the body part. Then I'd do that exercise for all I was worth and then next day, if the top part of the triceps, for example, was sore, I would jot that down in a little book (this book formed the basis for the second appendix in this book). Then the next time, I'd perform that same exercise with a slight variation — or a different one entirely — and then note what region of the muscle was affected.

I recommend that a person starting out or even someone who has been working out for a while, to perform three different exercises for the biceps. Here's the routine: Perform three sets of standing barbell curls, three sets of dumbbell incline curls and another three sets of high pulley bench curls.

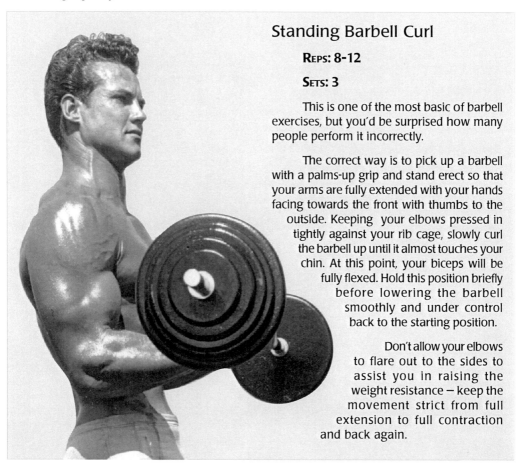

Standing Barbell Curl

Reps: 8-12

Sets: 3

This is one of the most basic of barbell exercises, but you'd be surprised how many people perform it incorrectly.

The correct way is to pick up a barbell with a palms-up grip and stand erect so that your arms are fully extended with your hands facing towards the front with thumbs to the outside. Keeping your elbows pressed in tightly against your rib cage, slowly curl the barbell up until it almost touches your chin. At this point, your biceps will be fully flexed. Hold this position briefly before lowering the barbell smoothly and under control back to the starting position.

Don't allow your elbows to flare out to the sides to assist you in raising the weight resistance — keep the movement strict from full extension to full contraction and back again.

Incline Dumbbell Curl

REPS: 8-12

SETS: 3

Sitting back on a 45-degree incline bench, take hold of two moderately-weighted dumbbells (they should be as heavy as you can handle in perfect form). With a smooth contraction, simultaneously curl up the dumbbells to the fully-contracted position and then lower them slowly, under control, back to the fully-extended or starting position. Do not swing the dumbbells up and, if possible, offset the weights on the dumbbells so that more plates are on the side closest to your thumb.

In other words, the outside of your hand should be jammed against the plates, and the remainder of the bar should be hanging down from the thumb side so that your biceps are not only under constant tension, but supinate naturally, due to the offset grip, at the top of the curl. Even if the dumbbells you use aren't adjustable, you can still offset your grip jamming your hand firmly against the inside plate closest to the little finger so that the majority of the dumbbell is hanging down the thumb side.

Start at the bottom from a straight or pronated position and then, as you curl the weight upward, slowly twist or supinate your palm, so that the outside of your hand is higher than your thumb at the top of the curl. You'll find — as I did — that this really works well.

Another device you may want to install on your incline curling bench is a "rear-stop bar." In back of the incline bench, you would put little rings through which would be placed a stop-bar (it can even be a cutoff barbell sleeve) which will, when properly affixed, serve to keep your arms stationary throughout the movement. This prevents you from swinging or cheating the weights up on this movement — either backward or forward.

When your arm is braced against the bar, your biceps — and your biceps alone — will be doing the work.

High-Pulley Bench-Curl

REPS: 8-12

SETS: 3

Place a bench under the high pulley, lie on your back facing the pulley. Grab the bar with your hands approximately one foot apart, in the thumbs-out position, making sure that the pulley is directly over your knees.

Keeping your upper arms in place, curl the bar to your chin with smooth movement. Repeat for three sets of 8 to 12 reps.

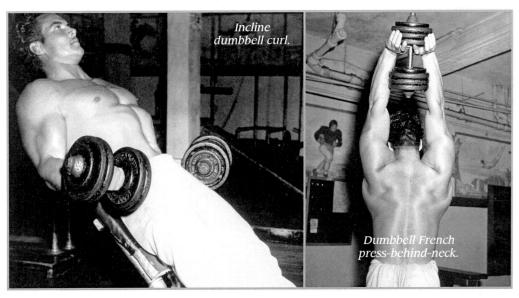

Incline dumbbell curl.

Dumbbell French press-behind-neck.

The Workout: ❺ Triceps

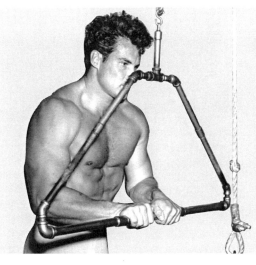

Press Down or Triceps Pushdowns
(bar, high pulley)

Reps: 8-12

Sets: 3

The first exercise to train your triceps that I would recommend is the high overhead pulley pushdown with your hands spaced about six inches, or a hands-width apart. The type of handle doesn't matter very much — I usually ended up with a straight bar but if it's slightly curved, that's okay, too. Sometimes it's actually more comfortable for your wrists if the bar is somewhat curved. Perform three sets of this movement.

Dumbbell French Press-Behind-Neck

Reps: 8-12

Sets: 3

Hold one dumbbell with both hands, your elbows right next to your ears. Keep your elbows in this position as you bend and straighten the elbows to raise and lower the dumbbell behind your head. Be sure to lower the dumbbell as far as you can to really get a good stretch and to ensure a full range of motion.

Triceps Extension Bench Press
(dumbbells)

Reps: 8-12

Sets: 3

Lying on your back on a flat bench, take hold of two dumbbells. Your grip should be such that your palms are facing in towards one another and the side of your hand should be pressing against the plate at the bottom of the dumbbell resulting in an offset grip.

Lower the dumbbells — with your palms still facing in — from a position of arms fully extended above your chest to a point just behind your ears. You can even just touch the top of the flat bench before raising the weight back up to the top again.

Remember to LOWER ONLY YOUR FOREARMS. Keep your upper arms stationary throughout the movement to ensure that your triceps and not your lats or pecs move the weight.

One-Arm Cross Over or Dumbbell Cross-Faces

Reps: 8-12

Sets: 3

A great movement to alternate from time to time with one of the above triceps exercises (I would sometimes substitute it for the curl behind neck exercise) — and one that really packs the beef onto the lateral head of the triceps.

Lying on your back on a flat bench, take hold of one dumbbell in your right hand and — with your upper arm remaining perfectly still — lower the dumbbell to your opposite shoulder and then, once it touches your deltoid, raise it back to the starting position.

Do full sets, alternating arms for 8 to 12 reps each before moving on to the next set, until you've completed three sets per arm. Again, the grip should be offset so that the outside side of your hand is pressed firmly against the plate at the bottom of the dumbbell handle.

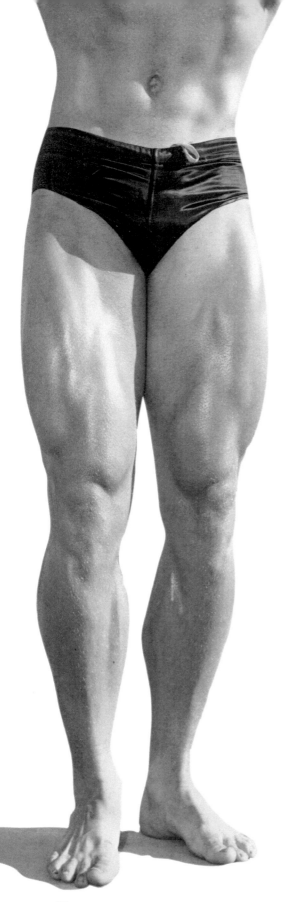

The Workout: ❻ Legs

Half Squat

REPS: 8-12

SETS: 3

When I was training hardest, I liked to perform what was then called half squats. Today they are referred to as parallel squats because your thighs end up parallel with the floor. And I used to use a very substantial stool when squatting. I would place the stool behind me — as it would be if I intended to sit down upon it — and then I would lower myself until my rear end just touched the stool and then return to the standing or beginning position of the squat. I wouldn't drop down and bounce against the stool because I knew that would be bad for my lower back, but I knew the stool was there and it really helped me to concentrate on the muscles involved in the movement.

Without the stool, you can't concentrate as much as you might think. I mean, are you parallel, are you above parallel, below parallel — how do you know for sure?

With a bench that is preset to the correct height, you don't have such worries; you just have to put a heavy weight on your back — 300 pounds or whatever is heavy for you — and just do it! Breath deeply, go down and just touch the bench and go up again. The bench serves merely as a gauge to let you know you've gone down far enough.

I'd recommend three sets of these. As a precautionary note, I recommend the use of a two-to-three inch block of wood under your heels for all types of squats. I never squatted on just the flat floor because it's bad for your knees and bad for balance. You need two to three inches under your heels.

"....When Steve Reeves first began showing interest in entering physique contests, he noticed that many of the contestants had very poor leg development in relation to their overall size. Steve concentrated on making his legs, particularly his calves, outstanding — and he did!"

— *Muscular Development, August 1967*

Hack Squat

REPS: 8-12   SETS: 3

The second frontal thigh (quadriceps) exercise is the hack squat or lift. You stand in front of a barbell. Bending down with your arms behind your body, grab hold of the barbell and stand upright so that the barbell is being supported at arm's length just behind the backs of your legs.

I used to wear a weightlifting belt and attached hooks to the back of the belt. The hooks would help support the weight of the barbell so I could concentrate more on the movement. I would go as deep as possible in the hack squat, making sure that the rear of my thighs compressed against my calf muscles.

Perfect style is important on all exercises, particularly with hack squats. Use as much weight as you can in perfect style so that all of your reps are executed smoothly up and down.

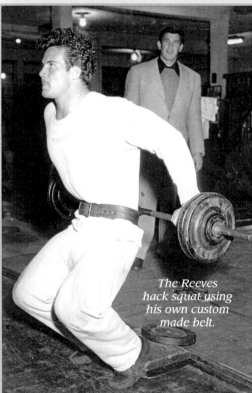

The Reeves hack squat using his own custom made belt.

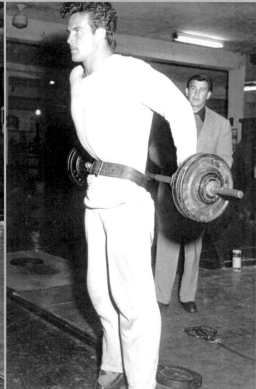

Front Squat

REPS: 8-12   SETS: 3

Like the hack squats preceding them, front squats target the lower frontal thigh muscles; however, they hit them on a slightly different angle. I would clean the barbell from the floor to my shoulders and perform the movement from start to finish with the barbell held in this position.

I never rested the bulk of the weight on my shoulders — easily 90 percent of the weight was supported by my palms.

Again, I recommend that you do no more than 3 sets on this movement.

Buddy-Assisted Leg Curl

REPS: 8-12   SETS: 3

To tackle the thigh biceps (hamstrings) on the rear of the thigh, I'd lie down on my stomach on a flat bench and my training partner would grab hold of my ankles and resist me as I curled my legs up towards my buttocks, and then use his body as resistance as I lowered my legs back to the starting position.

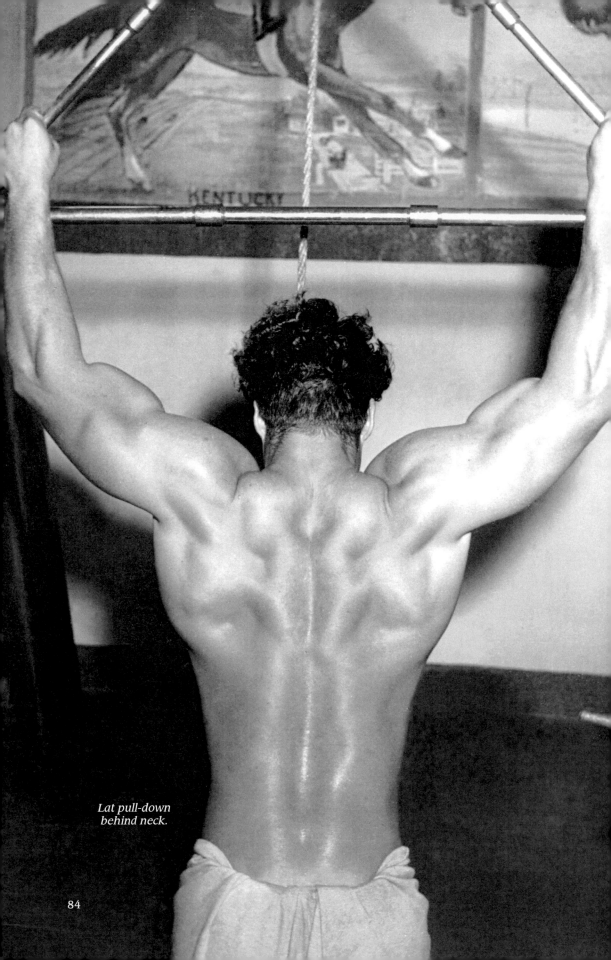
Lat pull-down behind neck.

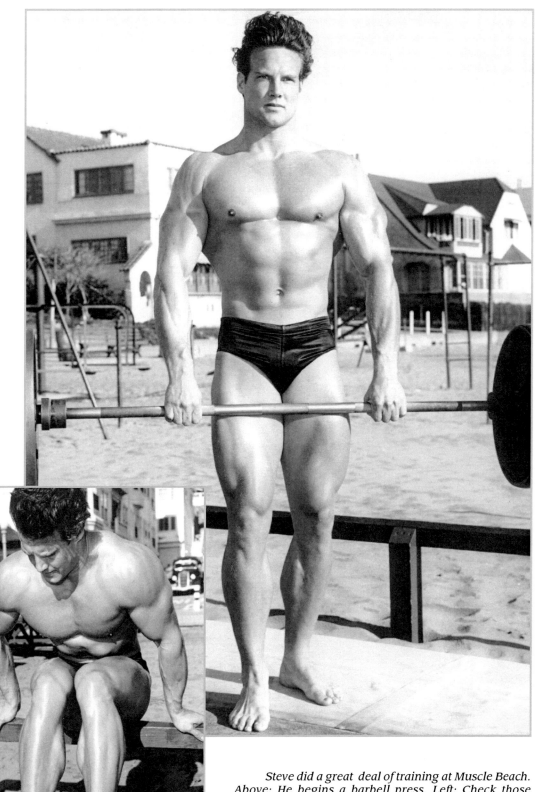

Steve did a great deal of training at Muscle Beach. Above: He begins a barbell press. Left: Check those beautifully developed deltoids and calves.

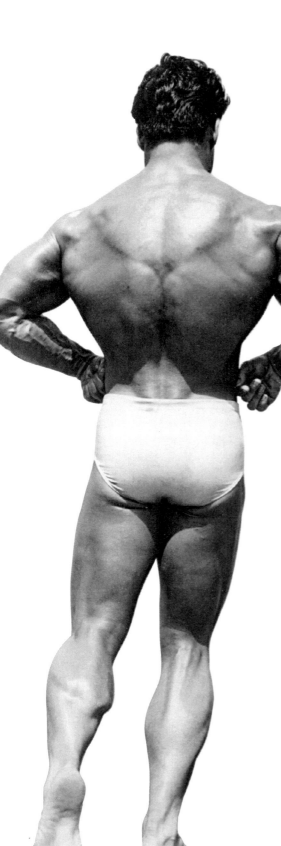

The Workout: ❼
Calves

Calf Raise and Leg-Press

Reps: 20

Sets: 1

I would always trained my calves on a leg press machine. It was the type of machine that had the resistance right above you. I'd lie under it and support the resistance on the balls of my feet.

I'd only do one set of 20 repetitions for my calves, going all the way up and all the way down.

I never hit my calves that hard because they were over 16-1/2 inches to start with and I didn't want them to grow out of proportion to my neck and arms. In fact, when I started my arms were only 13-1/2 inches — so I had to really concentrate on my arms more than my calves! My calves were up to 17-inches just through normal activity, but I got them up to 18-1/4 inches by training them hard.

The Workout: ❽
Lower Back

Good Morning

Reps: 8-12

Sets: 3

This great lower back exercise is seldom performed these days. It's called the Good Morning because it resembles bowing. It's also known as the forward bend.

I used to do deadlifts but I quickly switched to Good Mornings because deadlifts also work your glute muscles and I felt there was enough glute work in the squats. Also, I found that I derrived more benefit performing them while seated on a bench. Like most exercises, I strove to use as much weight as I could in perfect style and with a nice, easy cadence.

The Workout: ❾ Neck

Partner-Assisted Neck Flexion

Reps: 15 per side

Sets: 2, 1 per side

Utilizing the same buddy principle described above, I would also not neglect to train my neck.

Since no neck machines existed in those days, I would lie face up with my head over the end of a bench and my partner would provide resistance with his hands as I tried to move my head upwards. He would also provide firm and constant resistance to my head as I lowered my head back to the starting position.

I would then roll over so that I was on my stomach and lift my head backwards with my training partner providing resistance again on both the raising and lowering motion.

Remember, this routine should be performed only three days per week (i.e., on Mondays, Wednesdays and Fridays) for reasons that I've outlined elsewhere in this book. You may notice that I did not include any direct abdominal work in this routine. It's not that I'm against it (because I'm not — see Chapter 15, *Training the Midsection*), but I didn't feel I needed it because of all of the indirect effect the abdominals received from every other exercise I performed. For example, when I was doing triceps pressdowns, I found myself tensing my abs like crazy. Likewise for front squats — or any other type of squat — my abs always seemed to be getting a workout.

This routine evolved over time. I've tried different exercises, different ways but then I sat down and thought about my training logically and it occurred to me that, when you're working your muscles, you have to pump the blood to that area. And there's no use having the blood up in your deltoids and then doing some calf work next and then on to biceps and then back down again to the thighs — such a sequence just wasn't logical. It made far more sense to train the area where the blood already was, and that's how the sequence of shoulders, pecs, lats, biceps, triceps and then finally legs.

Some people believe that building the body is an art, others that it is a sport, and others think it's a science. My own opinion is that it is more of a science, and that's why the body must be trained in a specific sequence in order to obtain optimum results.

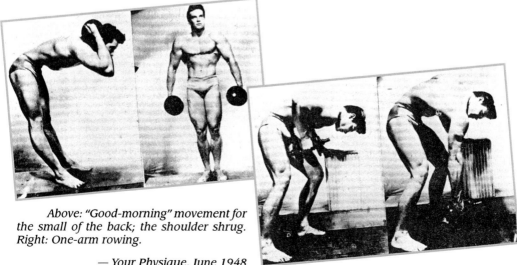

Above: "Good-morning" movement for the small of the back; the shoulder shrug. Right: One-arm rowing.

— *Your Physique, June 1948*

Chapter 15: Training the Midsection

The abdominals in the front and the obliques on the sides make up the midsection. When viewed by the athlete, this area often seems prone to overwork or neglect. I believe a proper perspective needs to be developed.

The abdominals need strength to ensure good health and physical fitness. Many people don't realize that chronic back pain is often caused by weak or undeveloped abdominals. The abs are a support structure that help maintain the internal organs, while contributing to the proper action of the muscles of the lower back, hips and thighs.

I have found that the very best exercise for good midsection fitness is the CRUNCH. This exercise strengthens the abdominals and helps trim the waistline. For an exercise to be most effective, the exercise must mirror the natural function of the muscle or muscle group being worked, and the crunch does exactly that. And best results are achieved when deep concentration augments the performance of this exercise.

Let's Get Crunching!

To do the exercise correctly, lie on a flat surface and bend the legs at a 90-degree angle. Place your hands on your forehead and inhale. As you begin curling the upper body forward and upward, keep your elbows pointing toward your knees while keeping your lower back on the flat surface. At the position of full abdominal contraction, exhale and hold the crunch in that position for a two count. Then begin inhaling as you slowly allow your body to return to the starting position. Repeat until you're no longer able to maintain perfect form.

The results of Steve's good midsection training.

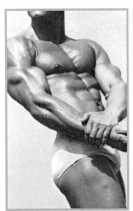
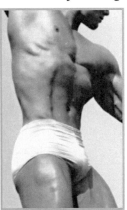
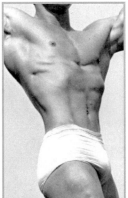
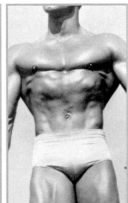

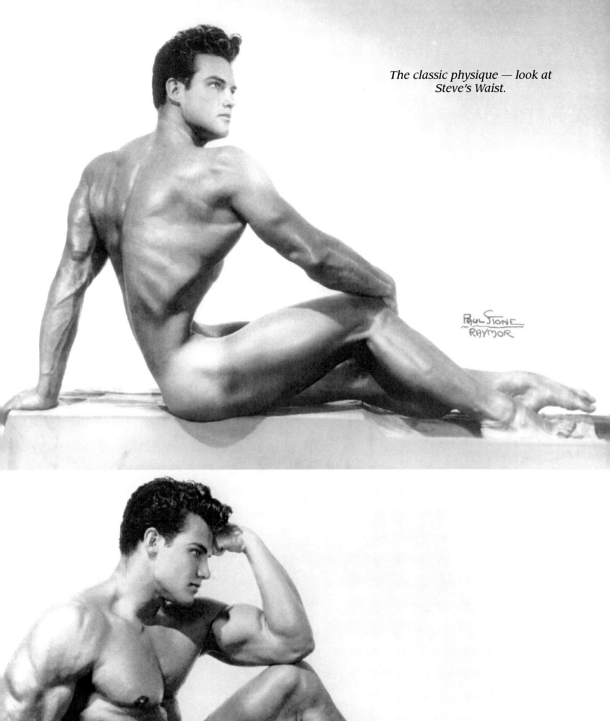

The classic physique — look at Steve's Waist.

Chapter 16: Maximum Muscular Development

For maximum muscular development use the maximum weight with which you are able to do 8 to 12 repetitions in good form with only 45 seconds rest between sets. By good form I mean that you should do each rep slowly and smoothly. Forget about bouncing or swinging the weight just to get it up. The weight should also move slowly and smoothly on the downward or eccentric half of the movement. Each exercise should be done through the full range of movement to the capacity of each specific joint.

Raising the weight should take approximately two seconds, lowering it three seconds. Most people neglect the negative or lowering portion of the movement. They let the weight just drop, with little resistance, instead of lowering it slowly and concentrating deeply on the muscle fibers being worked.

While doing each set, make sure that you don't stop until it's impossible to finish another rep in good form. I mean IMPOSSIBLE! The muscles being worked should experience momentary muscular failure somewhere between 8 and 12 reps. (If 8 reps are too hard, you need a lighter weight. If 12 reps are easy, you need a heavier weight.) Between sets, rest 45 seconds or the time it takes your workout partner to perform his set.

Then, for the next set, immediately lower the weight by 10 pounds or 10 percent and do another set of 8 to 12 reps until momentary muscular failure. Continue this until you've completed six sets for each muscle group. And so you won't get bored by repeating the same exercise over and over, you can do either of the following:

> Choose two different exercises for each muscle group and do three sets each.
>
> Do three different exercises and do two sets each.

On the last set of each muscle group, after you have pushed the last rep out and you can't do another one even if your life depended on it, you should immediately add weight to the bar or machine and do a set of negative only training. That means taking four to five seconds to lower the weight slowly.

At this point, you should have your workout partner or spotter help you raise the weight and then you'll repeat the procedure by taking another four to five seconds to lower the weight. Do as many "negative only" reps as you can until you are no longer able to stop the weight from descending. Your target rep goal should be 8 to 12 reps, depending on how slowly you lower the weight and how much weight you've added.

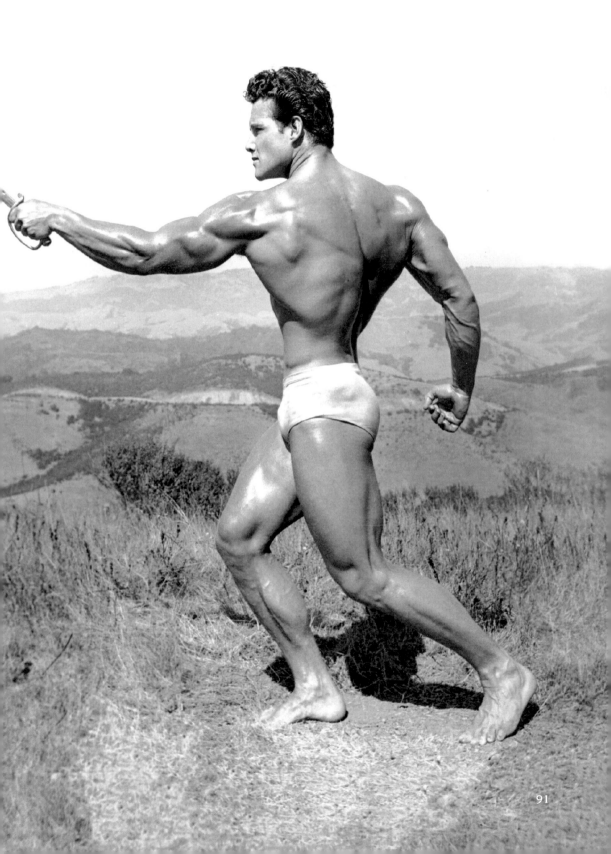

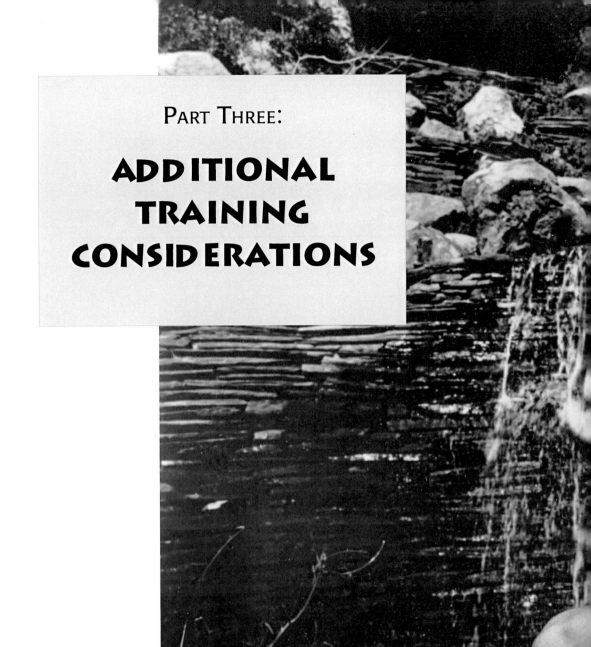

PART THREE:
ADDITIONAL TRAINING CONSIDERATIONS

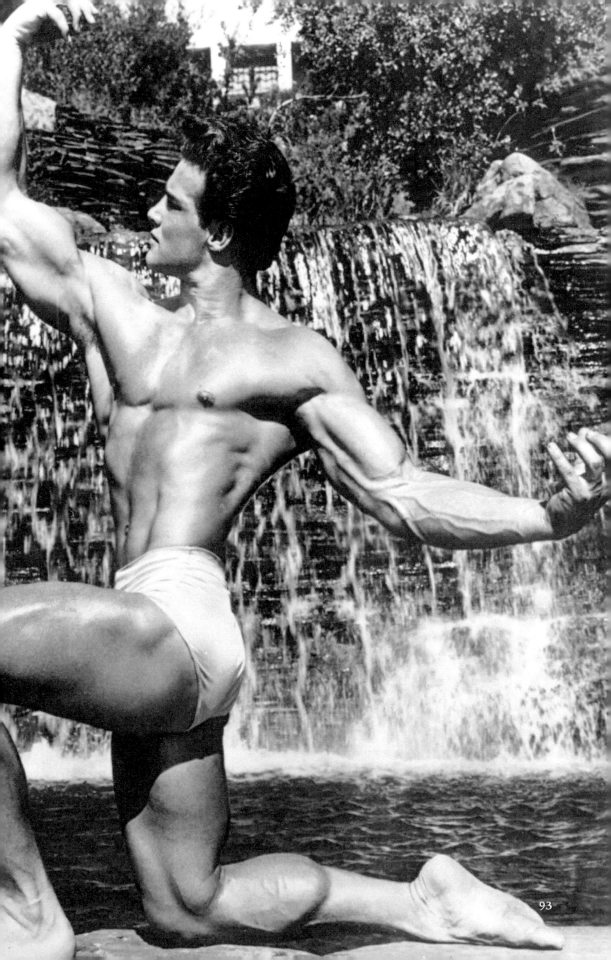

Chapter 17: Super High-Intensity Training

One of the most interesting aspects of bodybuilding is the abundance of techniques and nuances that will "kick start" your muscles into renewed growth. One of the most effective training techniques that I've ever encountered (and which I had cause to employ from time to time) is that of down-the-rack training.

Training "Down-the-Rack"

The down-the-rack system of training is performed as follows:

After warming up, start with the maximum weight with which you are able to perform an exercise in good style for 8 to 12 reps. For example, let's say that your maximum weight on the bench press is 250 pounds. Load the bar up to 250 pounds and work until you are no longer able to complete another rep.

Drop the weight by 15 pounds to 235 pounds and again work until you are unable to do another rep. Let's say you are able to do eight reps but are unable to complete nine; again drop the weight by 15 pounds to 220 pounds and continue working that muscle until momentary muscular failure.

Then drop the weight by another 15 pounds to 205 pounds and do as many reps as you can. Rest only 30 seconds in between sets or, if you prefer not to use a watch, rest only the time it takes you to get off the bench, change the weight and get back on the bench again.

Repeat this pattern of dropping 15 pounds until you complete six sets. If by dropping the weight 15 pounds each set you find it easy to do 12 reps, keep the weight as it is for the following set.

This chest workout is a sample of the Super High-Intensity Training System. Now select one exercise for each body part and perform it for six sets, in the same manner for a complete workout. Between muscle groups you can take up to a five-minute rest period.

A Sample Down-the-Rack Series

Warm-up, then start with your maximum weight (250 is an example; adjust according to your abilities):

Set	Weight	
1	250 lbs.	(maximum)
2	235 lbs.	(drop 15 pounds)
3	220 lbs.	(drop 15 pounds)
4	205 lbs.	(drop 15 pounds)
5	190 lbs.	(drop 15 pounds)
6	175 lbs.	(last set)

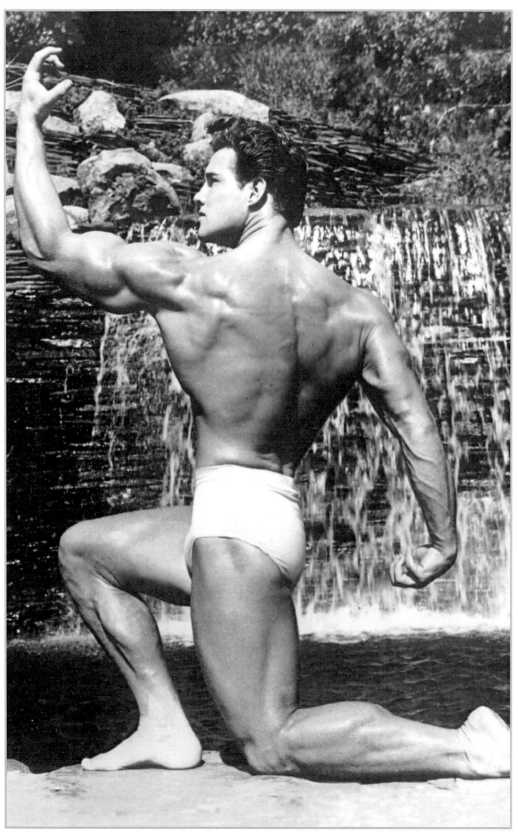

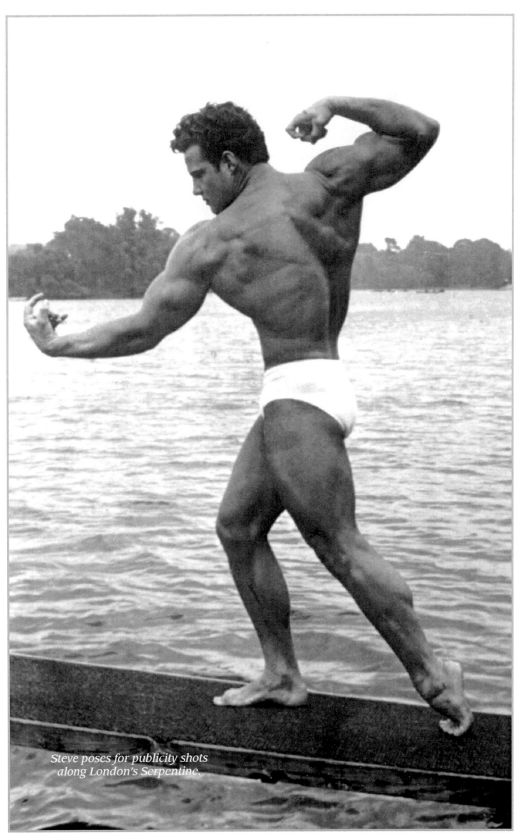
Steve poses for publicity shots along London's Serpentine.

Chapter 18: The Pyramid System

One of the more popular methods of training is the pyramid system, which has the trainee simply adding weight to each set he performs until he cannnot do more than three reps — then he decreases the weight.

For example, the trainee might start out with a warm-up of 190 pounds on the bench press and knock off 15 reps. After a 30-second rest, he would add 15 pounds to the bar, thus bringing his new total up to 205 pounds. With this weight, he would perform 12 reps and then rest for another 30 seconds. At which point, he would add 15 more pounds, bringing the weight up to 220 pounds, and perform nine reps with it. He would again rest for a period not exceeding 30 seconds, then add 15 more pounds to the bar, bringing it up to 235 pounds and continue for five reps.

As his starting level of strength has now diminished substantially, and as the weight has increased substantially, the trainee may at this point barely squeeze out three repetitions. Now he has reached the top of the pyramid — as high as he is capable of going for the day — and, after a one-minute rest, he'll reverse the pattern, dropping the weight, adding reps as he goes.

You can use this pyramid system to create a super high-intensity workout by selecting one basic exercise for each muscle group. You may want to refer to Appendix 2, "*My Favorite Exercises*," to help you with your selection.

Make 20-pound jumps when you are performing a multiple-joint movement using the large muscle groups such as the squat and the deadlift. On the leg press machine, take 25-pound jumps if that's the way the machine is set up.

While doing the bench press, I recommend you make 15-pound jumps. Other movements, such as curls, triceps extensions and laterals should jump only 10 pounds with each set.

Example: Course No. 1:

Press-Behind-Neck (wide-grip, barbell)

Bench Press (wide-grip, barbell)

Bent-Over Rowing (regular grip, barbell)

Standing Barbell Curl (regular grip, barbell)

Triceps Extension
(lying on bench, thumbs-in grip, barbell)

Squat
(parallel, with heels on a 2-inch block, barbell)

Deadlift (with knees bent, barbell)

Calf Raise (weight on knees, barbell)

Example: Course No. 2:

Upright Row (narrow-grip, barbell)

Incline Press (incline bench, dumbbells)

Seated Rowing (narrow-grip, low pulley)

Incline Bench Curl (incline bench, dumbbells)

Triceps Press Down (narrow-grip, high pulley)

Leg Press (strict form, leg press machine)

Forward Bend (seated on bench, barbell)

Calf Raises
(heels elevated on a 4-inch block, calf machine)

Chapter 19: Exercising in Opposition

Another highly effective technique to boost muscle growth and to keep things interesting, is the technique of exercising in opposition. That is, where you select one exercise for a specific muscle group and then follow it up immediately, superset style, with an exercise for its antagonistic muscle group. This technique guarantees balanced development and also results in some tremendous muscle pumps. Here are examples of some of the best exercises to be utilized in this system:

Exercises in Opposition
Opposing Pairs

Press Behind Neck (wide-grip; emphasis: deltoids and triceps) - with - **Pulldown Behind Neck** (wide-grip; emphasis: lats and biceps)

Upright Row (emphasis: deltoids) - with - **Parallel Bar Dip** (emphasis: pectorals and triceps)

Bench Press (wide-grip; emphasis: pectorals and triceps) - with - **Bent Over Rowing** (wide-grip; emphasis: lats and biceps)

Bench Press (narrow-grip; emphasis: pecs and triceps) - with - **Low Pulley Rowing** (emphasis: lats and biceps)

Incline Press (dumbbells; emphasis: upper pecs and triceps) - with - **Pulldowns in Front** (high pulley; wide-grip, emphasis: lats and biceps)

Supine Laterals (dumbbells; emphasis: pectorals) - with - **Bent Over Laterals** (dumbbells; emphasis: posterior deltoids)

Curl (barbell; emphasis: biceps) - with - **Triceps Extension** (high pulley; emphasis: triceps)

Parallel Squat (emphasis: thighs) - with - **Supine Knee Raises** (emphasis: abdominals)

Calf Raise (emphasis: calves) - with - **Toe Raise** (emphasis: shins)

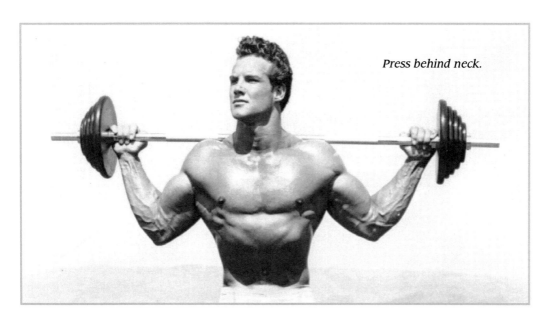

Press behind neck.

Leg Curl (emphasis: hamstrings on back of thigh)	- with -	**Leg Extension** (emphasis: quadriceps)
Back Raise (emphasis: erector spinae, lower back)	- with -	**Leg Raise** (emphasis: abdominals)
Forward Bend (emphasis: erector spinae, lower back)	- with -	**Sit-Up** (emphasis: abdominals)
Deadlift (emphasis: erector spinae, lower back)	- with -	**Alternate Supine Knee Raise** (emphasis: abdominals)
Pullover (emphasis: lats)	- with -	**Front Raises** (dumbbells; emphasis: deltoids)
Leg Press (emphasis: legs)	- with -	**Knee Raise** (vertical bench; emphasis: abdominals)
Shoulder Press (emphasis: deltoids and triceps)	- with -	**Chin-Ups** (emphasis: biceps)
Hack Lift (emphasis: thighs)	- with -	**Alternate Knee Raise** (vertical bench; emphasis: abdominals)
Front Squat (emphasis: thighs)	- with -	**Alternate Incline Knee Raise** (emphasis: abdominals)
Reverse Curl (emphasis: biceps)	- with -	**Reverse Triceps Extension** (emphasis: triceps)
Leg Adduction (emphasis: inner thigh)	- with -	**Leg Abduction** (emphasis: outer thigh)

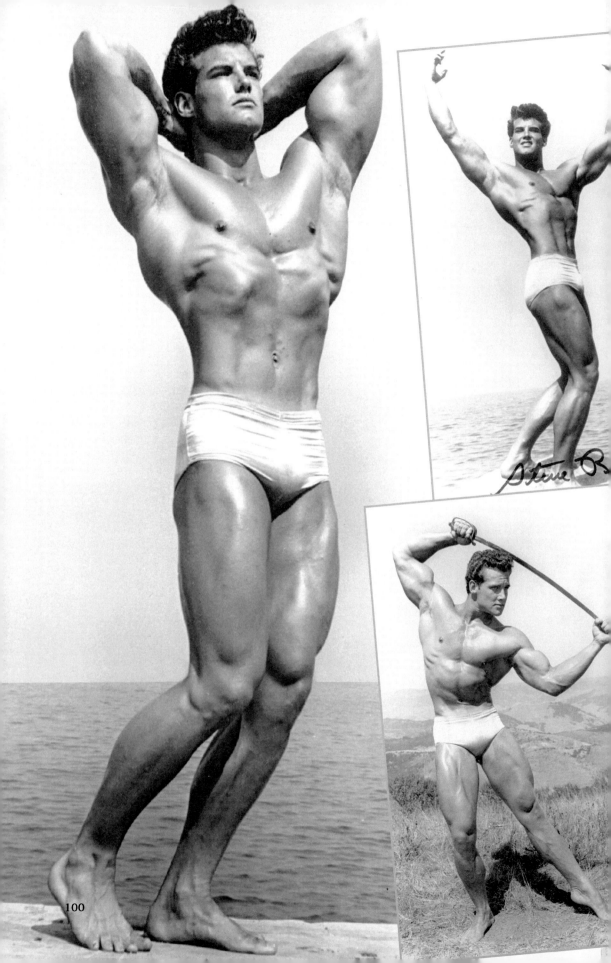

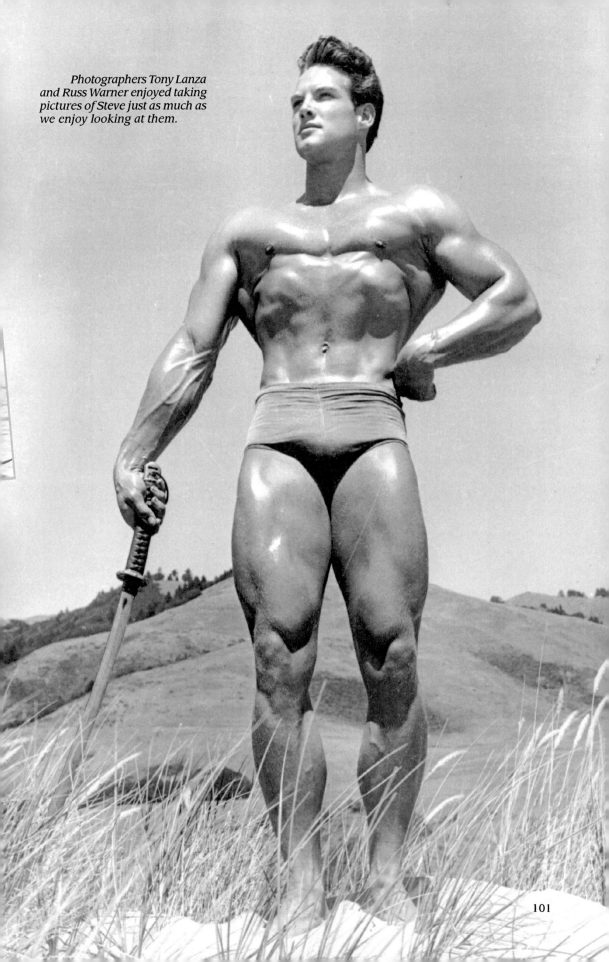

Photographers Tony Lanza and Russ Warner enjoyed taking pictures of Steve just as much as we enjoy looking at them.

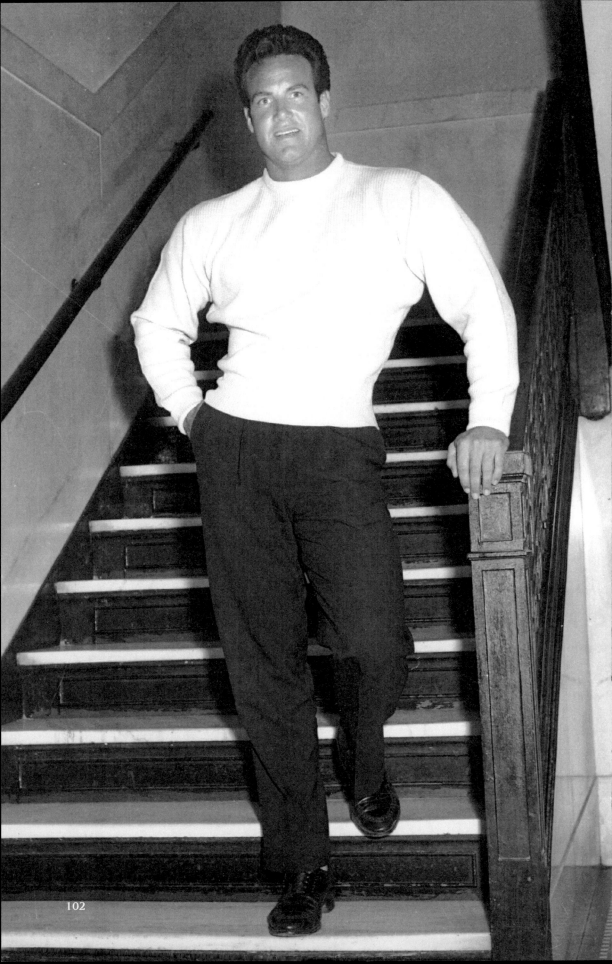

Chapter 20: Circuit Training for the Executive

This course is for those who want to tone up their muscles, improve their cardiopulmonary system, their endurance and possibly lose a few pounds, but who are limited as to the amount of time they can spend exercising.

After you have done a general warm-up and stretches, warm up with 20 repetitions of dumbbell swings. Gently swinging a light dumbbell between your legs, then over head and back. Then move on to your first exercise in the series:

UPRIGHT ROW
Muscle group emphasis: Shoulders
Repetitions: 12-15
Weight: Heavy as possible
Note: As soon as you complete these, rush to do a set of :

FORWARD BENDS
Muscle group emphasis: Firms and strengthens the lower back
Repetitions: 20
Weight: No weight on this exercise
Note: When you have finished these, without resting do a set of :

BENCH PRESSES
Muscle group emphasis: Chest
Repetitions: 10-15
Weight: Heavy as possible
Note: After you finish your bench presses, do a set of:

BREATHING PULLOVERS
Muscle group emphasis: Develops lung capacity
Repetitions: 20
Weight: 10 pounds
Note: As soon as you have finished the pullovers, do a set of:

BENT-OVER ROWING
Muscle group emphasis: Upper back
Repetitions: 10-15
Weight: Heavy as possible
Note: After these, immediately do a set of:

SIDE BENDS
Muscle group emphasis: Front and sides of waist
Repetitions: 20 per side
Weight: No weight on this exercise
Note: Upon completing your side bends, do one set of:

BARBELL CURLS
Muscle group emphasis: Biceps
Repetitions: 10-15
Weight: Heavy as possible
Note: When you have finished these, do one set of:

TRUNK TWISTS
Muscle group emphasis: Front and sides of waist
Repetitions: 20 reps per side
Weight: No weight on this exercise
Note: After you have completed these, do one set of:

TRICEPS EXTENSIONS ON THE OVERHEAD PULLEY

Muscle group emphasis: Triceps
Repetitions: 10-15
Weight: Heavy as possible
Note: After the these, do one set of:

BENT KNEE CURL-UPS

Muscle group emphasis: Waist
Repetitions: 20
Weight: No weight on this exercise
Note: Perform this exercise on a floor mat, rather than on a sit-up board, and immediately upon completion, do one set of:

SQUATS

Muscle group emphasis: Thighs
Repetitions: 10-15
Weight: Heavy as possible
Note: Upon completing your squats, do one set of:

BENT-KNEE LEG RAISES

Muscle group emphasis: Waist
Repetitions: 20
Weight: No weight on this exercise
Note: Upon completing the set, do one set of:

CALF RAISES

Muscle group emphasis: Calves
Repetitions: 20
Weight: Heavy as possible
Note: After completing calf raises, do one set (in each position) of the following exercise:

NECK EXTENSION AND CONTRACTION

Muscle group emphasis: Neck
Repetitions: 20 (in all four directions: front, back, left side, right side)
Weight: No weight in this exercise

Note: This concludes your workout.

In order to get the most benefit from your cardiopulmonary system and gain muscular size, tone and endurance, you must move from one exercise to another without resting. I have designed this course so that you do an exercise that tones and reduces the waistline in between the weight resistance exercises. This way, you will get a "breather" (so to speak!) between the more demanding exercises while still keeping your circulation and heart rate up to a desirable level.

When starting this exercise program, be careful not to over exert yourself. Check your heart rate every 10 minutes to make sure that you are not exceeding 75 percent of your predetermined maximum heart rate (or whatever limit your doctor recommends).

> You can figure your heart rate by subtracting your age from 220 — and then multiplying the remainder by .75. For example, if you are 50 years old, subtract 50 from 220 and then multiply by .75. (e.g.: 220-50 = 170 x .75 = 128 — therefore, your high-end target heart rate would be 128 beats per minute).

You can get excellent results at a lower heart rate too, depending on your fitness level. Some experts recommend starting off in the 60-percent or 65-percent range. Check with your physician before beginning any exercise program, and follow his/her advice regarding heart-rate levels.

Chapter 21: A Training Program for Seniors

The older man who comes to bodybuilding can expect some wonderful results. It's always recommended that you commence with a complete physical check up and regularly consult with your physician before beginning any form of resistance training but, assuming your doctor gives you a clean bill of health, you're going to love the benefits you will get from the program I'm about to outline for you in this chapter.

Start out with a good warm-up exercise such as Power Walking on a treadmill, (see Chapter 23 for more details on this incredible form of physical training), riding a stationary bike or working out on a Nordic Track, followed by some stretching exercises. (See Chapter 8 for information on stretching exercises.)

After you have finished your warm-up and stretches, you are ready to start on a progressive-resistance program using weights. You will discover that it is the best way to get in shape in the shortest period of time.

The method of progressive-resistance works as follows: Start out with a weight with which you are able to perform between 12 and 15 repetitions.

If you are unable to complete 12 reps while performing an exercise, lower the weight 10 pounds. If, on the other hand, you are able to complete 17 reps on an exercise, you are starting with too little weight and should raise the weight by 10 pounds.

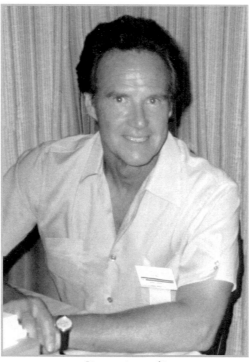
Steve, at age 60.

When you have gotten stronger on an exercise, and are able to do 16 repetitions, add 10 pounds. Start with 12 reps and work up to 16 reps before raising the weight again.

You will discover progressive-resistance will give you fast results if followed properly. When embarking on any new exercise program, it's always wise to start out easy and work up gradually to your potential. Don't put an increased demand on your body until it is ready for it. If in doubt, check with your doctor to see if you are in good health BEFORE you start on your way to building a healthier, more fit body.

Make a habit of stretching and doing a good warm-up and stretching before you engage in a sport or start your weight training program. When you are past the "half-century" mark, your joints, tendons and ligaments aren't as supple as they were when you were younger. I can't emphasize enough the importance of warming-up and stretching before you start your workout.

The Training Schedule

Exercise	Muscle	Equipment	Reps	Sets
Upright Rowing	Shoulders	Barbell	12-15	1
Standing Press	Shoulders	Barbell	12-15	1
Bench Press	Chest	Barbell	12-15	1
Bent-Arm Lateral	Chest	Dumbbells	12-15	1
Bent-Over Rowing	Back	Barbell	12-15	1
Pullovers	Back	Barbell	12-15	1
Standing Curl	Biceps	Barbell	12-15	1
Incline Curl	Biceps	Dumbbells	12-15	1
Press Down	Triceps	High Pulley	12-15	1
Supine Triceps Extensions	Triceps	Dumbbells	12-15	1
Leg Extension	Legs	Machine	12-15	1
Leg Curl	Legs	Machine	12-15	1
Forward Bend (seated)	Lower back	Barbell	12-15	1
Calf Raise	Calves	Calf Machine	12-15	1
Curl-Up (bent knee)	Midsection	No equipment	20-25	1
Leg Raise	Midsection	No equipment	20-25	1
Side Bend	Midsection	Dumbbell	20-25	1

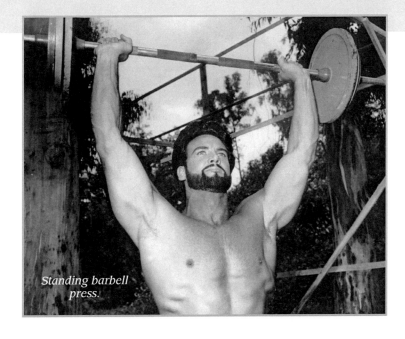

Standing barbell press.

Chapter 22:
Muscle Control — and the Art of Posing

Practicing muscle control improves the lines of communication between the brain and the muscle fibers being worked. This increases the efficiency and speed of muscle development and motor skills.

I believe it will be worthwhile for you to spend 10 to 15 minutes each day practicing muscle control. This can be done in one session or done several times a day for shorter periods. Spend twice as much time on the muscle group that you feel is not up to standards with the rest of your body.

Muscle control can be practiced while sitting in a chair, at a desk or table. To practice controlling the muscles of the calves, hamstrings, forearms, biceps, pectorals, lats and abdominals, do the following:

Sit in a chair with your lower legs placed at a 90-degree angle to your thighs. Rest your forearms on your knees. Focus on contracting one muscle at a time. Be sure to contract each muscle and release repeatedly for one to two minutes.

To practice controlling the deltoids, simply sit in a chair, lean forward and rest your head and forearms on the top of a desk or a table. Keep your head resting slightly above your hands, which will be in the palms-down position.

Controlling the quadriceps is easy: Simply rest your legs in the outstretched position on top of a desk or another chair or footstool.

To practice controlling the triceps, place a chair facing away from your desk or table. Extend your arms behind your back and rest them on the table or desk. Again, concentrate on one muscle, contract and release it repeatedly.

Posing—The Art of Physique Display

Let's talk for a moment about how you prepare yourself for posing and how you choose your poses. First of all, you should choose your poses from looking at how the pros display their physiques in the photographs in bodybuilding magazines. You might, for example, note that a certain bodybuilder looks very impressive in a particular lat pose. So you check yourself out in the mirror to see how that pose complements your physique. If you're lucky, you'll look at least as good and dramatic as the guy in the

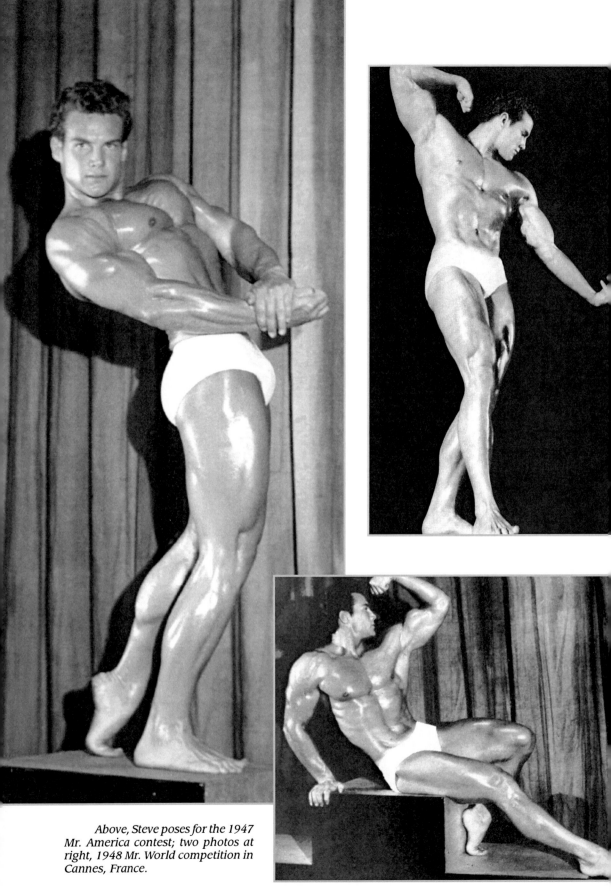

Above, Steve poses for the 1947 Mr. America contest; two photos at right, 1948 Mr. World competition in Cannes, France.

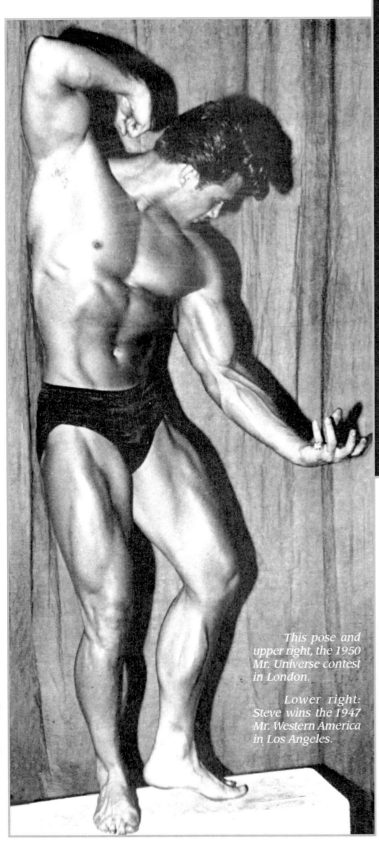
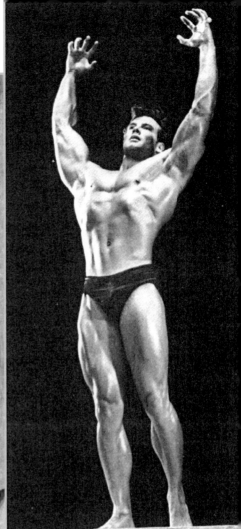

This pose and upper right, the 1950 Mr. Universe contest in London.

Lower right: Steve wins the 1947 Mr. Western America in Los Angeles.

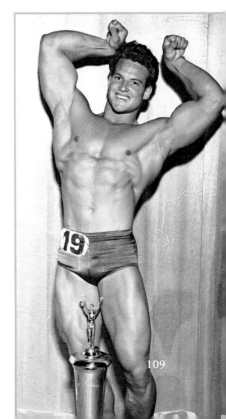

magazine. If not, you'll at least learn which poses do NOT suit your particular body type.

When I was preparing for bodybuilding contests at Yarick's Gym, there was a great big skylight at one end of the gym. There were also mirrors on either side of the gym walls. At a certain time of the day, usually around 10 a.m. or 2 p.m., we discovered that the lighting was ideal for posing. So we would come in on Sundays, and oil up a little bit, stand under the skylight and check our poses in the gym mirrors.

Sunday would be our experimental posing day. All of the bodybuilders who had a contest coming up would each try out some new poses that we'd seen bodybuilders demonstrate in the magazines, and then we would coach each other from the sidelines about how we could make these poses work more effectively for us. "Twist more to the right," one fellow would shout. "Lock your back leg," another would call out, and, by doing so, we learned the subtle nuances of physique presentation.

Posing was different in those days — at least as far as the lighting at contests went. Back when I competed, the lights were slightly overhead at perhaps a 70-degree angle to the stage. It gave us more shadows when we were in the spotlight, with the shadows augmenting our separation and detail.

These days the guys go out on the stage and it's really well lit, perhaps too well lit at times, which occasionally results in many physiques getting "washed out" in the glare of the lights. Certainly the old-fashioned lighting made for a more dramatic effect. One good thing about the modern lighting is that the bodybuilders today can jump on the stage and they can be within six to ten feet from the center of the stage and they're still "on." The lighting is so broad that it's almost impossible for them to miss it. In my time, we had about eight inches to maneuver in, and if you were off by even three inches, that could make all the difference in the world as to how your physique would be perceived by the judges.

In any event, it must be remembered that everyone possesses a unique assemblage of physical attributes in addition to an individual personality and temperament. A posing routine, to truly be effective, must complement these attributes and at the same time express the essence of your personality. The style of posing you adopt will serve as a complete expression of you.

In selecting your poses, first assess your physical structure. In my own example, I would always determine what was my "best" or most dramatic pose — and then try to leave the audience (and the judges) with that as my last shot. I mean, you know you have to hit the compulsory poses of side chest, side triceps, front and rear double biceps and front and rear lat spread. But somewhere amongst all of those poses is one — or a variation on one — that will be your best pose.

Recognize that pose and practice it to perfection. Doing so just might win you a major contest some day.

I used to close my posing routine with the arms extended overhead "lat" pose that appears on the cover of this book. Famed Hollywood producer, Cecil B. DeMile called it "Perfection in the Clouds," and it surprised me to learn that he had a giant blowup photograph of it in his office. Nevertheless, this only serves to underscore the absolute value in learning what your best pose happens to be.

I would conclude my routine with that pose as a way of saying "Thank you," to the audience for their positive reaction and support, and also to leave a strong visual impression on the judges who still had to watch other competitors go through their poses. It truly was my signature pose, and the only other bodybuilder I've seen who could do this pose effectively was the great Sergio Olivia.

The first time I ever saw that pose was in a picture of Alan Stephan. Alan had great lats and was, in fact, Mr. America the year before I won it. He did this pose and he did it very well. And, from looking at that picture, I decided that I would like to try it and see if it would work for me. Fortunately it did, but it really underscores the need to experiment and to look at the magazines or attend contests and see what poses the top bodybuilders are hitting.

Putting It All Together

While recognizing your "best" pose is important, putting together an impressive routine, complete with graceful and fluid transitions is also critical.

I used to start my posing routine with a lat shot. After I'd completed this pose (I'd hold it for two to three seconds for maximum effect), since my arms were already out to the side, I would flow smoothly into a double biceps shot. From the front double biceps pose, I could make a fluid transition into a three-quarter back shot. Again, I would hold this pose for effect, and then slip into a side triceps shot. This is just what I would do, but you may find that this doesn't work for you. In that case, just do whatever comes smoothly to you so that you look graceful instead of clumsy when you're posing on stage.

Why I Never "Pumped Up"

I never did any type of pumping up before my posing routine. I found by working at the gym and then looking in the mirror afterward, that if you pump up and try to do a pose, you shake. Your body trembles — which looks awful to the judges — and you also lose some of your definition. So instead of looking relaxed and dynamic, the man who pumps up like crazy before his posing routine ends up looking strained, shaky and not nearly as well cut. No matter how much my competitors would pump up at a contest, I would only do a few stretches just to limber up, but I would never do any pumping up.

Augmenting Through Posing

To really bring out a muscle group when posing, you have to know the degree to which it can be contracted and still be visually striking. Sometimes a maximum contraction will hinder — rather than help — you in your efforts to display a muscle group to its fullest potential. You can also do little tricks to augment the muscle's appearance. For example, when executing a three-quarter twisting back pose, you want to make your waist look as small as possible, and you want to twist just enough to make your back look as broad as possible. If you twist too much, you get too much back in the pose and not enough waistline — and you've lost your taper. Conversely, if you don't turn enough, you don't get enough back in there, and again, you lose your taper and width. It has to be right on.

The same holds true with hitting a side chest pose; getting your arm in the right place is the key to its impact. If your arm is pulled too far back, as some bodybuilders do, you'll look like you have a large chest but a small arm. If your arm is too far forward, it will look like your arm dwarfs your chest. So you've got to find that "sweet spot" in between — which only comes from practicing your posing — and learning to position your arm in just the right place to show both a thick, muscular arm and a broad, muscular chest. My best pose, in this respect, was with the triceps down and tensing the abdominals at the same time. That way I was able to display both the abdominals and the chest.

Also, when hitting a front double biceps pose, if you draw your arms too far back, you won't be able to reveal much in the way of taper or lat development. And if you hold your arms too far forward, your lats will flare out nicely but your arms will be at the wrong angle to look impressive. Again, practice your posing in front of a full-length mirror and see which angle works the best for you.

Posing is not easy. It's very difficult, as you have to be fully aware of angles, lighting and conditioning. You have to isolate which muscle group you're going to be flexing and really concentrate on bringing it out and displaying it to its fullest potential — while not relaxing any part of your body.

I actually posed on stage maybe 12 times in my whole life, which consisted of six contests and six exhibitions — which isn't much on-stage experience. But knowing the above factors saw me through to victory nearly every time.

Ending with a couple more shots from the 1950 Mr. Universe contest in London.

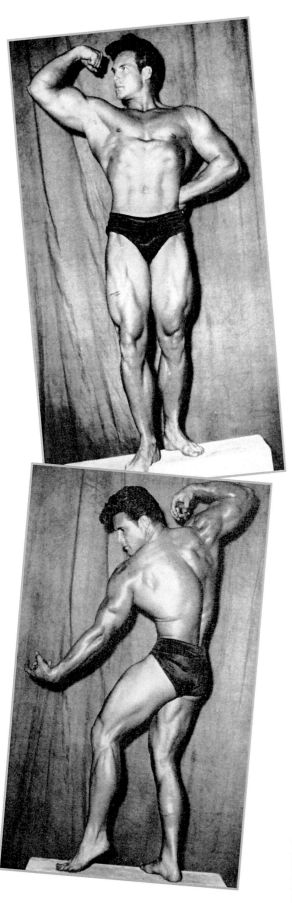

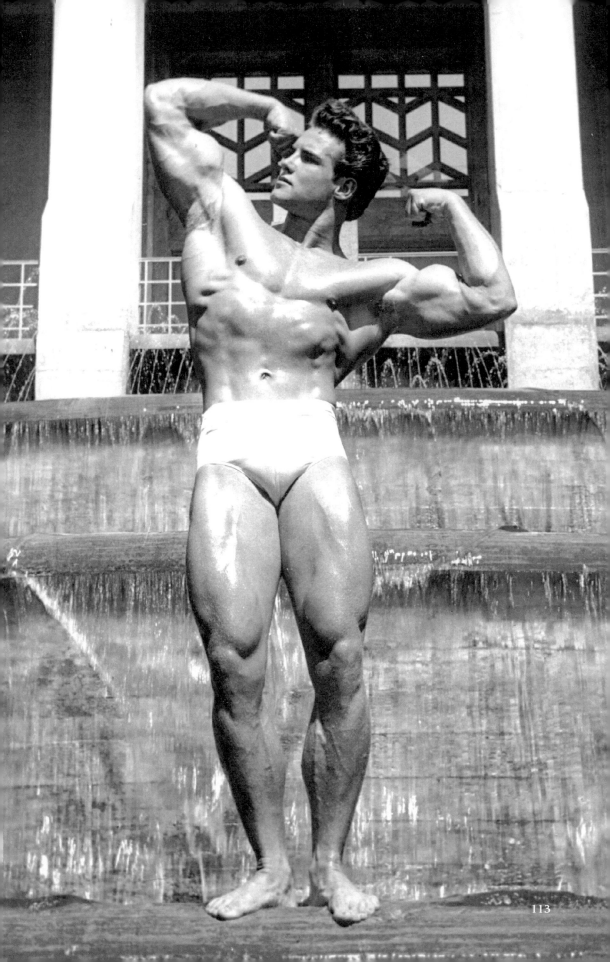

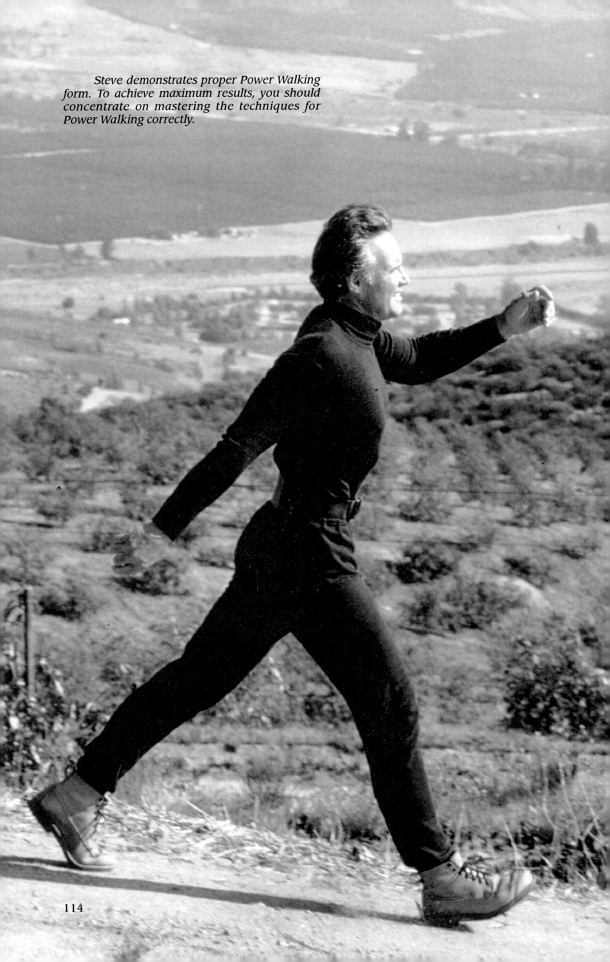

Steve demonstrates proper Power Walking form. To achieve maximum results, you should concentrate on mastering the techniques for Power Walking correctly.

Chapter 23: The Power of Walking

The majority of bodybuilders and other strength athletes have a great deal of anaerobic energy enabling them to perform at a high intensity level for a short period of time. They look healthy and strong and muscular, yet they lack one thing — the aerobic capacity to run, swim and bike for an extended period of time. In other words, many of these big muscular guys lack endurance and get tired in a hurry.

On the opposite end of the pendulum are the aerobically-trained athletes such as long-distance runners and marathoners who have a high degree of cardiopulmonary fitness, but don't have that strong, healthy muscular look. In fact, the majority of world-class marathon runners look emaciated.

One of the reasons for writing this book is to outline to you the ways to combine these two extremes — aerobic and anaerobic exercise — to help you look fit, feel fit, think fit, be fit and stay fit.

The known sports that combine aerobic and anaerobic conditioning to a somewhat balanced degree — building that strong muscular look and muscular endurance, along with a high degree of cardiopulmonary fitness — are distance rowing, distance swimming and cross-country skiing. These sports use all of the major muscles in the body, at a fairly high degree intensity, for an extended period. Thus, they fulfill the three requirements for true fitness: muscular strength, muscular endurance and cardiopulmonary fitness.

Most people don't have easy access to a lake or river to practice rowing. And in most places, the weather doesn't permit year 'round training. Distance swimming also requires a river, lake or Olympic size swimming pool in which to train. Cross-country skiing is limited to the cold climates and winter months. All of which makes it a seasonal sport in northern states and limited to high elevations (if found at all) in the southern climate zones.

As a very effective alternative to these superb conditioning sports, I have developed an exercise which you can do year 'round, in any kind of weather, regardless of where you live. I call it the POWER WALK.

The ancient Greeks believed a long walk was a tonic. Famed entertainer/songwriter, George M. Cohan prescribed a walk to banish dejection and despair. "You never heard of anyone," he said, "doing away with himself after a long walk." Former President Harry Truman, known around the world for his evening sojourns said, " I believe walking will allow me to live longer."

Regardless of the time period or the personality involved, "the best of all exercises" as

Thomas Jefferson called it, has always been walking. Yet the Greeks in their wisdom did not know the precise physical effects of walking.

Today's doctors know well the benefits of brisk walking and are quick to expound on them. Says the American Medical Association's Committee on Exercise and Physical Fitness: "Walking briskly, not just strolling, is the simplest and also one of the best forms of exercise." Adds noted heart specialist, Dr. Paul Dudley White, "It is the easiest for most individuals, one that can be done without equipment except good shoes, in almost any terrain and weather and into very old age."

It is with this in mind that I developed a logical extension of the brisk walk; I call it the "Power Walk." The Power Walk is walking with a progressive resistance. You see, ordinary walking can build heart and lung capacity only to a certain extent. Beyond that, the walker must go on to something more strenuous. I have therefore carried the exercise one step further, with the progressive resistance principle, as it's more difficult to walk fast than slow, more difficult to walk five miles than one mile, more difficult to walk on a six-percent grade than one level grade, and it's more difficult to walk with 20 additional pounds on your body than just your body weight. In essence, these are the factors that distinguish the Power Walk from any other variety.

My development of the Power Walk came about rather casually through training of my Morgan horses. While leading a group trail ride across the Borrago Desert, the riders and myself would get off our horses and walk beside them for 10 minutes out of each hour. During the 10 minutes of walking, I found that I had some difficulty keeping pace with my horse, Banner, whom I had trained to walk fast. After lengthening my stride and breathing rhythmically, I found it was much easier to keep pace with him. But I was still being left behind so I started swinging my arms vigorously in opposition to my leg movements, and found that I was able to keep up. At the end of 10 minutes, I noticed that I was a good quarter mile ahead of everyone else! While waiting for the others to catch up, I recounted what I had experienced and thought, "This is a terrific aerobic exercise!" I realized that I had just worked every muscle in my body.

This was the exercise I had been looking for all of the years I was an actor. It is virtually injury-free and supplies the needs of a total fitness program. With some experimentation and practice, I developed Power Walking.

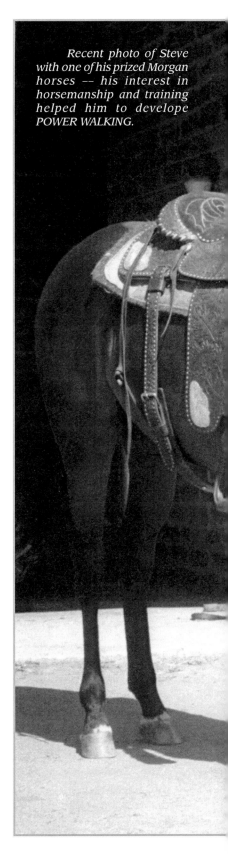

Recent photo of Steve with one of his prized Morgan horses -- his interest in horsemanship and training helped him to develope POWER WALKING.

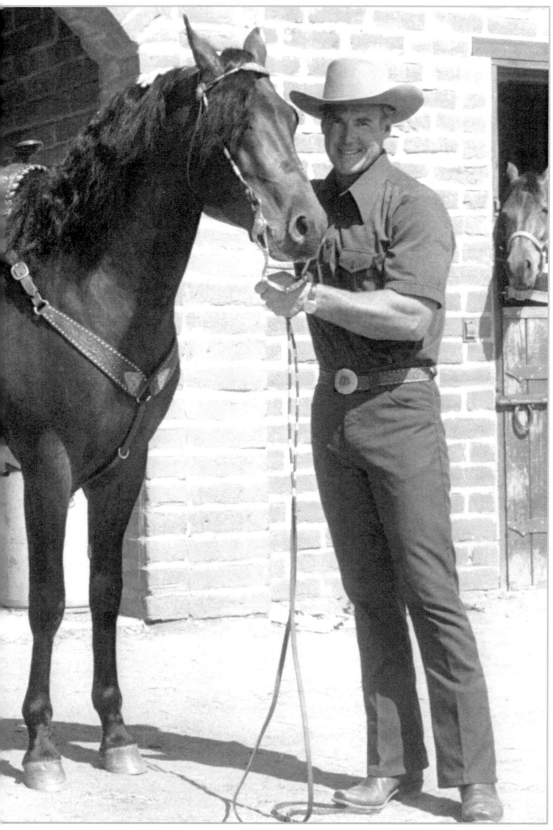

There are, in fact, many benefits of this newly discovered method of walking that became immediately apparent to me. I found that I was breathing more deeply, that my heart had picked up a few beats, and that I wasn't sore the next day because the walking had increased my circulation so much that it had removed the lactic acid in my body.

I further learned that if I breathed in for three paces and out for three paces, I had more endurance and seemed to get the right amount of oxygen at the right time. When walking uphill, I modified the breathing pattern so I would breathe in every two paces, then out for two paces.

As you might have guessed by now, breathing is very important in the Power Walk. You should breathe in semi-Yoga fashion. In other words, in three stages: upper, middle and lower. Your lower is the most important because it's your lower lungs, the powerhouse of the Power Walk. To breathe properly—this is vital—expand your ribs down by your waistline. Rhythm is very important in everything you do in life, so keeping a rhythm as you do your Power Walk is essential. The rhythm of your arms, legs and breathing together gets you more attuned to the universe. Simply stated, the Power Walk consists of six key factors. They are:

1. Length of stride	4. Degree of incline
2. Speed of movement	5. Amount of weight carried
3. Distance traveled	6. Rhythmic breathing

Put Pep in Your Step and Pride in Your Stride

A person looks much younger with a long, springy stride. As people grow older, their stride tends to become short and choppy, giving them the appearance of old age, when in fact, that may not be the case at all. A long stride stretches the muscles in the legs. Muscles that are long, look better and work better for you because they are loose. Lengthening your stride is the most important thing to remember as you begin doing the Power Walk.

When you feel you have perfected your stride, begin thinking about adding speed by changing your cadence and making it faster and faster.

I recommend that you start out by walking approximately a half mile at a speed that is comfortable for you. Concentrate on the fact that you are exercising and be aware of your breathing. Soon it will become automatic, just like driving a car. Fitness can be fun, and to get the most enjoyment and benefit from it, be aware of all the factors that will help you get the greatest benefits.

Then, as you progress to a half mile at a brisk pace, you should start to set goals for yourself. In the beginning your goal should be to reduce your walking time for the half mile to eight minutes.

Remember, your initial fitness level may give you the impression that you'll never be able to walk at that pace. Don't get discouraged. You didn't get out of shape overnight and you won't get back in shape overnight, either. Be patient, you've taken the most critical step — the first step! You've recognized the need to be more physically fit and you've identified the most effective means to achieve your ultimate goal — Power Walking!

Once you can walk a half mile in eight minutes, start walking a mile. I recommend doing it in 20 to 30 minutes to start. Gradually increase your speed until you can walk a mile in less than 14 minutes, if you are 5-feet-6-inches or shorter, and in 12 minutes if you are 5-feet-7-inches or taller. At this point, you are doing what I call the pure Power Walk.

Working Harder

After you are able to do a pure Power Walk, you can increase its intensity three ways: You can walk a longer distance, select a course that has hills, and carry additional weight while you are walking.

Taken in progression, each factor increases the demand on your body and its systems. At first you may wish to use only one of the three methods. But eventually you will be using all three. To continue to improve, you need to use all three. What is more important, you will want to use all three.

Start with adding hills to your course, thereby increasing the resistance. After you've walked on a course with hills and can maintain your five-miles-an-hour pace, add weight.

The first type of weight I recommend using are hand weights. I got the idea of using hand weights for Power Walking one day when I was walking on the beach and saw two interesting-looking rocks the size of baseballs. I decided to take them home for my collection. When I picked them up and began walking with them, I immediately discovered that it felt good to have something in my hands as I walked, to counterbalance the thrust of my legs. They probably weighed no more than two pounds each.

Shortly thereafter, I developed my own weights for Power Walking that are adjustable from one to five pounds. I personally use the five-pounders. Naturally, anyone starting out should begin with the one-pound weights and build up to three, four or five-pound weights (depending on your body weight), after six months to a year of doing the Power Walk.

I like to put the major portion of the added weight around the waist. I have devised a belt that is weighted with shot which can be adjusted to various weights. The midsection is where the human body can naturally carry the most weight, just above the hip bones, so it is a perfect place to add weight in exercising. Backpackers can carry 40 to 50 pound sacks on their backs because the weight is distributed between the shoulders and the midsection with the use of a belt around the waist. I believe that a person can work up to 10 percent to 15 percent of his/her bodyweight in added weight. I would distribute up to 10 percent around the waistline and five percent using hand weights. I also like ankle weights. However, use those only after you've become accustomed to hand and waist weights.

I arrived at the extra weight distribution by trial and error. I tried using 10-pound weights with my hands, but found that I couldn't get the same swinging movement with my arms or the same length of stride. Stride is the last thing I want to cut down because it's one of the most important factors in Power Walking. So five pounds is really the maximum for each hand weight.

The same held true on the waist weights. I went up to 15 percent of my bodyweight on the waist weights, but found that my stride was being diminished by this. So, I cut back to 20 pounds around the waist, 5 pounds in each hand, 2-1/2 pounds around the ankles and a pair of shoes that weighed two pounds, thus giving me about 20 percent of my bodyweight.

A person really has only to dedicate 30 minutes a day, four days a week to Power

Walking. Actually, it isn't so much a dedication as it is preventive medicine. If you spend some time exercising each day and aren't sick that year, then you're happier and healthier and you're even ahead financially, because you didn't have to take sick time off from work.

After you have done the Power Walk for six months to a year, depending on your age or fitness level, you should be able to carry 10 percent to 15 percent of your bodyweight around your waist and in your hands. For example, if you weigh 200 pounds, you should be able to carry 20 to 30 pounds of extra weight. And if you can go five miles, at five miles per hour with 15 to 20 percent extra weight, then you are what I call not just FIT, but SUPER FIT!

In Power Walking, as in any other sport, you get your second wind. You find that as you're walking along, it will become difficult to continue. Then, your breath will come again and you'll feel like you're in overdrive. When you are truly in shape, mountains seem like hills, the hills seem level and level feels like going downhill.

Get in Shape, Stay in Shape

To get in shape, walk two to three miles. To stay in shape, walk one to two miles. It is important to keep a log book of your progress. That way you can note the number of miles traveled, the amount of time it took, whether the course had inclines, and the amount and type of extra resistance weights you carried.

Time is not a real problem with any form of exercise. It took many people 30 years to get out of shape, so why should they expect to get into shape in 30 days? You can burn up to 300 calories in just 30 minutes of Power Walking. If you walk an hour or two a day, this can take off well over one pound of fat a week.

If you lose one pound of fat a week for 20 weeks, you've lost 20 pounds. After all, it took years to put on that extra weight. Be patient. It's much better for your body in general, especially your skin, to lose the weight gradually. This will help ensure that the weight loss is fat and not lean muscle and you have a far better chance of keeping it off for good! The good news is that it's not going to take years to take it off!

Most people are only 10 to 20 pounds overweight. By using the Power Walk and eating a well-balanced and nutritious diet, you can easily get in shape. Walking has the added advantage of exercising the whole body and almost all of your muscles — especially if you get a rhythm going and swing your arms freely. In fact, many people simply need to redistribute the weight they already have, or, in some cases, add a few pounds.

And there are other physical benefits. Your bones are shaped and levered to absorb shock. Furthermore, each one of the bones, ligaments and muscles in the foot are exercised while walking. So are the leg muscles from the ankles to the hips.

As you Power Walk, the leg muscle contractions compress the veins, improving the return of blood from the lower extremities. This blood must flow back to the heart — mainly against the pull of gravity. When you improve the muscles of your legs, you are also improving the pumping action provided by these muscles, thereby improving circulation.

Power Walking is the most natural exercise there is. You can do it from the cradle to the grave. You don't need any expensive equipment, just a comfortable pair of shoes. And it is extremely low risk. Perhaps most importantly, you can Power Walk even if you're not in good overall physical condition.

Any exercise where you are putting out energy and effort will strengthen your heart,

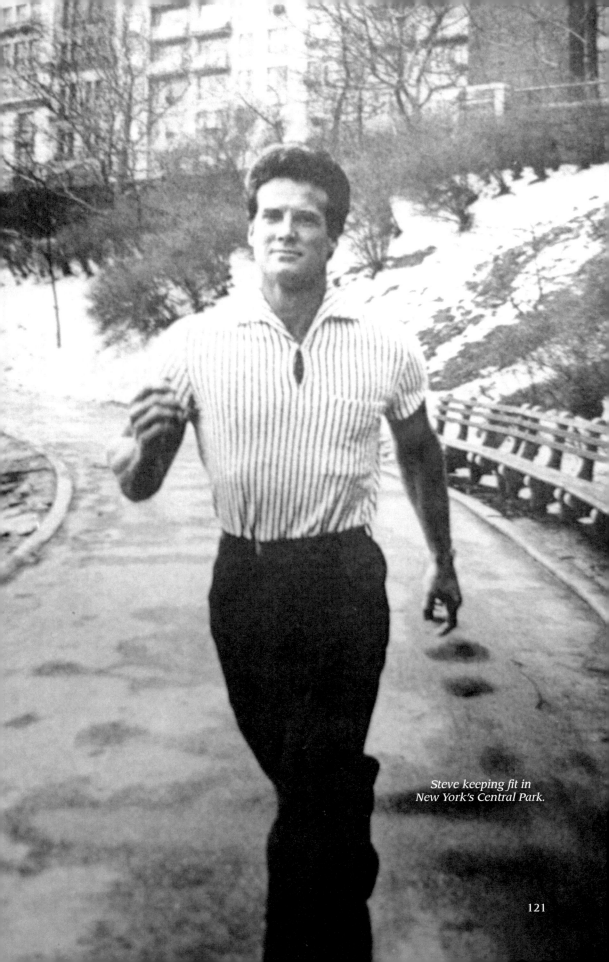
Steve keeping fit in New York's Central Park.

thereby making it a stronger pump. All the breathing you do and the rhythm being employed will increase the size of your rib cage — that means a bigger chest — and the increased oxygen intake will put more red corpuscles into your blood, making you healthier and more energetic.

By cutting down the time it takes you to walk a half mile or increasing the distance from one mile to two miles, you get a tremendous feeling of accomplishment. The Power Walk improves your posture by helping you walk erect.

I have a friend who had been jogging off and on for a number of years. I put him on the Power Walk and he hasn't stopped since. He is able to maintain a consistency without any strain to his cardiovascular or pulmonary systems, and he loves it. Toning your cardiovascular system and burning extra calories requires that you to use big muscles. I'm talking about those below the waist, which represent 75 to 80 percent of your total muscle mass. The Power Walk does this.

Power Walking Isn't Jogging

How does the Power Walk differ from its first cousin, jogging? In many ways. First, you are much less likely to get injured doing the Power Walk. It was discovered that many joggers are developing what is called "jogger's knees," experiencing a tightening of the Achilles tendon and finding that their lower backs are getting out of shape from pounding the pavement so much.

This cannot happen with the Power Walk, because it's the most natural exercise available. A person who has difficulty jogging, will not have the same problems with the Power Walk. You can expend the same amount of energy without being prone to injury. And the Power Walk is better psychologically because it's a positive exercise.

Jogging causes you to use only about 35 percent of your aerobic capacity. If you were giving jogging your all, you'd be sprinting or doing something like the 100-yard dash! With the Power Walk, if you're giving 95 percent of your capacity, you're not holding yourself back or doing a different form of the exercise.

What many people fail to realize is that with jogging, you purposely hold yourself back because you know that you have to jog so many miles or so many minutes, which would be very difficult if you were giving 100 percent of your energy 100 percent of the time. With the Power Walk, you can go 95 percent. With your rhythmical movements, your arms and legs working, your arms swinging like pendulums, you are constantly renewing your oxygen and energy as you go along. You don't incur an oxygen debt. In other words, you take in as much oxygen as you're using.

The breathing aspect is what will help you achieve success with the Power Walk because it sets the pace of the rhythm for you. To this day, nobody has come up with a walk that's really different. The race walk, for example, requires lessons to learn and it certainly isn't graceful.

The Power Walk is especially good for women. When a woman jogs or runs, the breasts tend to shrink due to the constant bouncing and breakdown of the tissue. Whereas walking is a steady, brisk movement that actually helps firm up tissues.

The Power Walk is a great conditioner too! You'll look and feel better. I want to give you something that's going to make you look better, feel better and be better. You will be in firmer shape. Just remember, a man can weigh 175 pounds and look good or bad. It's primarily a matter of conditioning. It isn't how much you weigh. It is the quality of your body.

Physical benefits aside, the Power Walk relieves any tension and anxieties you may encounter during the day, whether they're from work, family, relationships or anything else. If all anxieties and tensions are relieved, you can think more clearly. I get many good ideas when I'm on my walk. And when I get home, I jot them down. Study the lives of many great writers and artists and you will discover that much of their most creative thinking came during those times when they were walking and close to nature. I like to feel that I am following the dictates of William Cullen Bryant, who a century ago said, "Go forth, under the open sky, and listen to nature's teaching."

Poets and philosophers, in discussing the virtues of walking, have persisted in their belief that it provides a sense of self-renewal. When returning home after a brisk walk, you feel tired, yet, in a positive and tranquil way. Your tiredness is indeed, satisfying, almost as if you've given your entire body a transfusion.

Naturally, as with anything new, the person entering the Power Walk program should first check with his or her physician, explain the program and get the physician's approval. You must be sure that you are in good enough physical condition to begin a new exercise program, even though the Power Walk is the most natural of all exercises.

And while it may not be natural for the businessperson to jog down the street on the way to work, it is very natural for him or her to be able to walk briskly down the street. So put some power in your walk. It's something that truly can be taken in stride!

Power Walking - The Great "Bun Burner" for Women!

I am often times asked about exercise programs for women who do not wish to build excessive muscle, yet would like to get as physically fit as possible. The best advice I can give in a situation like this is to have them seek out a program that would effectively tone the many different muscle groups, aid in fat reduction, and give good aerobic benefit.

As an actor in Europe, I was often on location, which considerably hindered my personal exercise program. As a result, I came to depend on running as a means of staying in shape. However, there were many obvious disadvantages to the up and down jarring action. Due to an ankle injury I suffered during my last film, I was forced to seek other forms of exercise, as I could no longer use running to maintain fitness.

Fortunately, through riding and training my Morgan horses I was able to discover the benefits of brisk walking and with some experimentation and practice I developed the Power Walk. With the development of Power Walking, I could see how it would be especially beneficial for women. It develops and firms the hip area (the glutes) and doesn't have the jarring effect jogging does.

When Power Walking, it is very important to use the heel-to-toe technique, but not in the traditional sense. The heel of the advancing foot should touch the ground with your knees slightly bent. As you roll to the flat foot position, straighten your leg and drive it forcefully to the rear with your buttock muscles.

It is extremely important to use the glutes as the driving force when pushing your leg to the rear. This is where the "bun-burning" effect, as I call it, comes from. As your front leg is driven back, the opposite leg should be thrust forward, taking as long a stride as possible. Always push with the buttocks and not the toes. When these leg positions are practiced and done properly, you have accomplished the first step in Power Walking.

To obtain maximum benefit from Power Walking, swing your arms back and forth in a pendulum-type motion in opposition to your leg movement. Your arms should swing forward to an approximately 45-degree angle and back to approximately 30-degrees. Your left arm should swing forward as your right leg moves forward. When practicing this, you should allow your arms to hang in a relaxed position.

As you begin, it may seem a bit awkward at first, but soon it will feel as natural and comfortable as any exercise you may now be doing. One of the most important things to remember when Power Walking is to lengthen your stride. A long stride will stretch your leg muscles and make them more flexible. As these muscles stretch, they will look better and more importantly, they will feel better. They will be less prone to aggravation and injury such as pulls, strains and tears.

Rhythmic Breathing

Another stage in using Power Walking as a fitness program is breathing. As with any form of exercise, breathing properly is vital to obtain maximum benefit. Once you have practiced your stride and become comfortable with the arm movement, you should concentrate on breathing properly.

The particular form of deep breathing I recommend is rhythmic. The rhythmic breathing I have found to work best is to inhale deeply for three strides (right, left, right) and then exhale forcefully for three strides (left, right, left).

Rhythmic breathing involves three different stages, through the lower lungs first, then the middle lungs and finally the upper lungs. I believe the stage in which air is drawn from the lower lungs is the most important since most people are generally shallow breathers and use mostly the upper portion of their lungs during respiration. As a result, they use their lower lungs less than the middle or upper region.

In the first phase of the three-stage rhythmic breathing technique, you should try to push your abdomen outward as this will enable you to force air to flow into your lower lung area. In the second stage, you should attempt to expand your lower ribs and middle thorax areas to bring air into the middle portion of your lungs. The third stage involves arching your chest outward, and at the same time drawing your abdomen inward to support your lungs. This will enable you to bring the maximum amount of air into your upper lung area, thus allowing you to fully exercise your total lung area.

When exhaling, force air should out with the same technique, only in reverse. I would like to emphasize the importance of the distinct stages flowing smoothly from one to the other.

As with the other aspects of Power Walking, your rhythmic breathing will quickly feel very natural so that you can now focus your attention on all the nuances of the Power Walk.

Dramatic Results

Nothing can give you "instant fitness," but I can assure you that within one month of Power Walking three times a week for at least 15 minutes a session, you will see and feel dramatic results!

Power Walking increases oxygen intake and improves your circulation. Your body has nearly 60,000 miles of blood vessels, mostly capillaries, that bring oxygen to your muscles. Only a few of these capillaries are open when your muscles are not in use. Nearly 50 times as many will be open when your muscles are involved in exercise. When you Power Walk, the muscle contractions compress the veins, thereby improving the return of blood from the lower extremities. This blood must flow back to the heart against the pull of gravity. When you improve the muscles in your legs, you also improve the pumping action of these muscles. As a result, your total body circulation is improved.

Another fantastic aspect of the Power Walk is that it can improve posture. When you Power Walk, you walk erect. You don't lean forward. Your shoulders are laid back, but not forced back. The muscular tone provided, as well as the time spent concentrating on postural alignment will do nothing but help your posture.

Since Power Walking enables you to develop all-around fitness, it is also a valuable conditioner for any activity that involves physical exertion. Many of my friends love to hike. Using the Power Walk has helped condition them for the long treks. I feel Power Walking is also a great conditioner for weekend athletes — people who plays tennis or golf on the weekends, but need something during the week to help them maintain an optimal level of fitness.

It isn't terribly difficult to see how changes in our daily habits over the years have adversely affected our level of fitness. To a large extent, the automobile has made walking obsolete, while television has replaced our more strenuous pastimes. As the pace of life seems to grow more hectic, junk food and fast food serve as quick-fix substitutes for good, well-balanced, nutritious meals. Time is the enemy. Convenience is the ally. Why take time to fix a good meal when a burger and fries can fill you up?

In many cases, our choice of conditioning activities are almost as counterproductive as our daily living habits. Everyone seems to be looking for a gimmick or fad—the easy way. In response to this demand, everywhere you turn there is a new diet, exercise gimmick or conditioning tool—anything to make us look younger, thinner, sexier, bigger, smaller or better. Few people seem satisfied with approaching their health in a scientific manner. No matter how bad the economy, people will always find a way to afford the luxury of beauty.

Truth be told, there is no quick fix. There is no miracle way to fitness or weight loss. But there are good and practical ways to achieve a firmer and more shapely body. These principles will not and have not changed.

When you practice and use the techniques I have explained here, you can look forward to the incomparable feeling of total fitness, because not only will you look great, you will feel great!

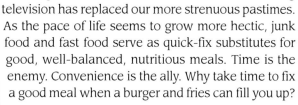

Steve Reeves trekked miles in "Sandokan the Great" released in 1964 — his movie roles demanded true fitness.

Week	Distance	Time Allowed	Extra Weights
3 Times per week minimum	in miles	recommended guidelines in minutes	H=hand weights W=waist belt A=ankle weights

Program 1:
For a 175-Pound Man 29 Years of age or Younger

Week	Distance	Time	Extra Weights
1	1/2	6-10	H-1 lb.
2	1	12-15	H-1 lb.
3	1	12-14	H-2 lb.
4	1	12-14	H-2 lb. W-5 lb.
5	1½	20-25	H-2 lb. W-5 lb.
6	1½	20-25	H-3 lb. W-5 lb.
7	1½	19-24	H-3 lb. W-5 lb.
8	1½	19-24	H-3 lb. W-10 lb.
9	1½	18-23	H-4 lb. W-10 lb.
10	1½	18-23	H-4 lb. W-15 lb.
11	2	25-32	H-4 lb. W-15 lb.
12	2	25-32	H-4 lb. W-15 lb. A-1 lb.

Program 2:
For a 175-Pound Man 30 to 50 Years or Age

Week	Distance	Time	Extra Weights
1	1/2	7-11	H-1 lb.
2	1	14-18	H-1 lb.
3	1	13-17	H-1 lb.
4	1	13-17	H-2 lb. W-5 lb.
5	1½	21-26	H-2 lb. W-5 lb.
6	1½	21-26	H-2 lb. W-10 lb.
7	1½	20-25	H-2 lb. W-10 lb.
8	1½	20-25	H-3 lb. W-10 lb.
9	1½	19-24	H-3 lb. W-10 lb
10	1½	19-24	H-3 lb. W-15 lb.
11	2	26-33	H-3 lb. W-15
12	2	26-33	H-3lb. W-15 lb. A-1 lb.

Program 3:
For a 175-Pound Man 50 Years of Age or Older

Week	Distance	Time	Extra Weights
1	1/2	8-12	H-1 lb.
2	1/2	8-10	H-1 lb.
3	1/2	7-11	H-1 lb.
4	1	15-20	H-1 lb.
5	1	15-20	H-2 lb. W-5 lb.
6	1	14-19	H-2 lb. W-5 lb.
7	1	13-18	H-2 lb. W-5 lb.
8	1½	22-27	H-3 lb. W-5 lb.
9	1½	22-27	H-3 lb. W-10 lb.
10	1½	21-26	H-3 lb. W-10 lb.
11	1½	20-25	H-3 lb. W-10 lb.
12	1½	20-25	H-3 lb. W-10 lb. A-1 lb.

Program 4:
For a 135-Pound Woman 29 Years of Age or Younger

Week	Distance	Time	Extra Weights
1	1/2	8-11	H-1 lb.
2	1/2	7-10	H-1 lb.
3	1	15-19	H-1 lb.
4	1	14-18	H-1 lb. W-5 lb.
5	1	13-17	H-1 lb. W-5 lb.
6	1	12-16	H-2 lb. W-5 lb.
7	1½	22-26	H-2 lb. W-5 lb.
8	1½	21-25	H-2 lb. W-5 lb.
9	1½	20-24	H-2 lb. W-7½ lb.
10	1½	19-23	H-2 lb. W-7½ lb.
11	1½	18-22	H-3 lb. W-10 lb.
12	1½	18-22	H-3 lb. W-10 lb. A-1 lb.

Program 5:
For a 135-Pound Woman 30 to 50 Years or Age

Week	Distance	Time	Extra Weights
1	1/2	8-12	H-1 lb.
2	1/2	8-10	H-1 lb.
3	1	17-21	H-1 lb.
4	1	16-21	H-1 lb.
5	1	15-20	H-1 lb.
6	1	15-20	H-1 lb. W-5 lb.
7	1	14-19	H-1 lb. W-5 lb.
8	1	13-18	H-1 lb. W-5 lb.
9	1½	23-28	H-2 lb. W-5 lb.
10	1½	22-27	H-2 lb. W-5 lb.
11	1½	21-26	H-2 lb. W-5 lb.
12	1½	21-26	H-2 lb. W-7½ lb.

Advanced Power Walking Programs

Here are five sample advanced Power Walking programs. Select the program that fits your age group and adjust the program as needed through personal trial and error. For more complete charts showing programs for men and women of different weights and ages — read my book "PowerWalking."

Chapter 24: Getting Smart about Nutrition

I've been an ardent practitioner of physical fitness ever since I was a teenager. Over the years, I've learned how to gain muscle, how to lose body fat and how to alter my body size and shape almost at will. This knowledge came in handy when I was making movies, allowing me to assume whatever the necessary physical proportions were required of the character I was to play — from Hercules to Morgan the Pirate!

When I played the title role in *Hercules*, for example, the producer of the movie wanted me to weigh no more than 210 pounds — all of it muscle. When I played the role of a cowboy in my last film, *A Long Ride From Hell*, I was required to reduce my weight to 190 pounds in order to fit the director's perception of how the character should look. My knowledge of both nutrition and exercise enabled me to achieve both of those looks.

I recall one time that I gained some unwanted weight. An injury to my shoulder required surgery, with the result that I was laid up for almost six weeks. When I was able to recover sufficiently to exercise, I combined a well-balanced, reduced calorie diet with regular exercise sessions, and those unwanted pounds quickly vanished.

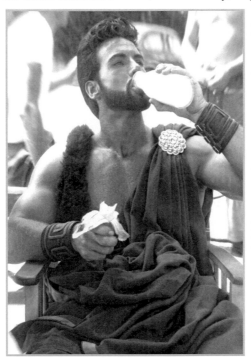

No matter how busy he was, Steve always ate healthy and nutritiously.

That's the real "secret" to keeping in shape. You don't need any special pills, "new" diets or, more recently, surgery — to alter your body fat stores and to control your weight. You need exactly what I just mentioned: a program based on equal parts of exercise, proper nutrition, logic and discipline.

The first step required to control your bodyweight begins and ends with what you put into your mouth. When you eat or drink too many products that contain calories, you gain weight. However, when you consume less than you need, you lose weight. And if you eat within the confines of your needs once your weight is normal, your weight will remain stable. The most important aspect regarding nutrition, however, is that you make sure that you're consuming a well-balanced diet.

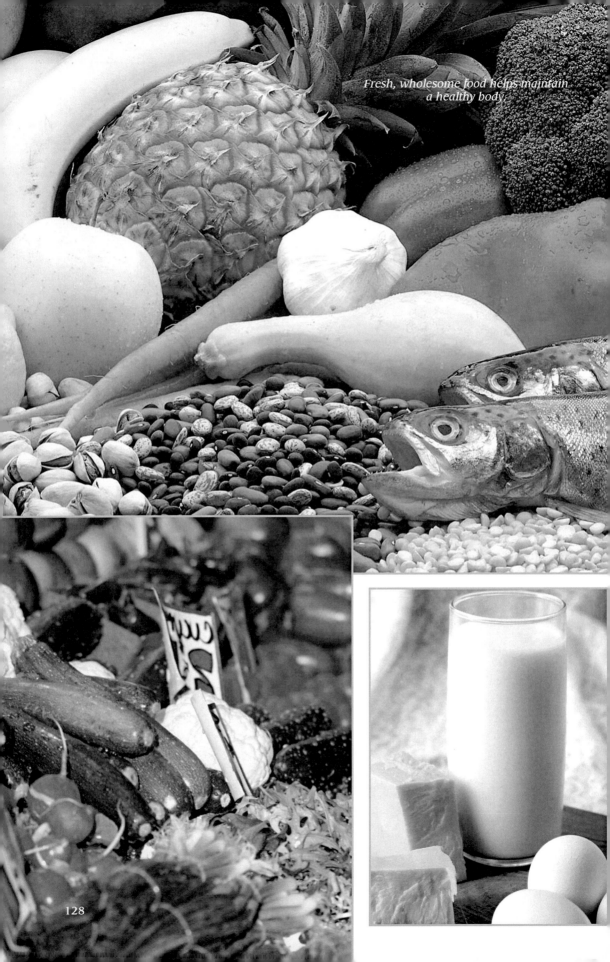
Fresh, wholesome food helps maintain a healthy body.

A Well-Balanced Diet

In addition to calories, each food contains nutrients — six groupings of bodybuilding ingredients that are absolutely essential for life. Remember that no one food contains all of the nutrients that your body requires to function optimally. Since every nutrient has a specific function in your body, a combination of nutrients is needed to make up a well-balanced diet. If you consume a nutritionally poor diet, you will eventually become ill. In fact, a nutritionally imbalanced diet could — in extreme cases — lead to death. The actual nutritional needs vary among individuals but every individual requires adequate portions of the following six nutrients:

Protein

Proteins have been called the fundamental building blocks of life. The word protein is derived from a Greek word meaning "of first importance." Proteins are composed of carbon hydrogen, oxygen, nitrogen and sulfur. Protein is necessary to build and repair body tissue, but some proteins are better than others for this purpose. A complete protein contains the essential amino acids in the most useful proportions and will best build and repair tissue. The best proportioned proteins are found in such foods as egg whites, milk, meat, fish, cheese and poultry.

Plant proteins are not as complete — these are found in grains, legumes (such as beans and peas) and nuts. You will have to eat large quantities of these plant foods in order to supply the body with usable protein. For those of you who prefer to get the major part of your protein from a non-meat source, I would recommend complementary food combining in which you consume foods that complement, or complete, one another in terms of amino-acid balance.

Amino acids are your body's building blocks. Although there are more than 20 amino acids, only eight are considered essential because they must be present in appropriate amounts to make up a complete protein. They are: tryptophan, phenylalanine, lysine, methionine, valine, threonine, leucine, isoleucine.

When you combine a food like beans — that is high in lysine but deficient in methionine, with wheat, that has an abundance of methionine but is deficient in lysine, you get more complete protein utilization. (For more information on food combinations, I recommend that you pick up a copy of *"Diet for a Small Planet,"* by Frances Moore Lappe.)

Carbohydrates

Carbohydrate foods are the major source of calories for people all over the world. They make up 50 to 60 percent of the American diet, and in other countries the percentage is even higher. They are easily digested and constitute the cheapest form of food energy. They are composed of carbon, hydrogen and oxygen. They exist as complex sugars and starches which are converted through digestion to simpler sugars which the body can utilize for energy. Carbohydrates include cellulose, which is important for roughage in the digestive tract. All carbohydrates eventually become glucose, a simple sugar which travels through the bloodstream and serves as a source of energy for the body tissues. Important carbohydrates are sugars, starches, syrups and honey. Carbohydrates are major constituents of vegetables, fruits, breads and cereals.

Fats

Fats are compounds of fatty acids and glycerol — another complex structure of carbon, hydrogen and oxygen — insoluble in water and greasy to the touch. The different fats in various foods help give the food its particular flavor and texture. Fats are especially important because they produce more concentrated energy — almost 2-1/2 times as much as protein or carbohydrates. They have a high satiety value in that they take longer to digest than other nutrients and therefore keep us from experiencing hunger for longer periods of time. Fats also carry the fat soluble vitamins — A, D, E and K. Vegetable oil, butter and margarine are the concentrated fats. Most meats and salad dressings, along with eggs, milk, mayonnaise and nuts have considerable fat, plus protein and/or carbohydrates.

Minerals

Minerals are found in foods mixed or combined with proteins, fats and carbohydrates. Calcium and phosphorus give rigidity to the bones and teeth. Milk is a good source of both. Minerals are also needed for normal blood clotting and proper functioning of the nervous system. Iron is a mineral essential in the diet because a lack of it can produce anemia, leaving us tired and listless. Meat and enriched bread are good sources of iron. Other minerals are essential to help maintain a normal acid-base balance in the body and other important functions.

Vitamins

Vitamins are complex organic compounds found in the foods we eat. They perform specific vital functions in the cells and tissues of the body. Called accessory food factors, they are needed for normal health, including good eyesight, strong teeth and bones, freedom from infection and disease, normal functioning of the nervous system, tissue respiration and other functions.

Water

Water is also essential to life. It is a necessary constituent of digestive juices and of every cell of the body. Approximately two thirds of the body's weight is water. It is a major component of blood, lymph and other secretions of the body, and helps regulate body temperature. As a carrier, it aids digestion, absorption, circulation and excretion. Moisture is necessary for the functioning of every organ of the body. Most foods contain a large percentage of water. You can live longer without food than you can without water.

Given the importance of these nutrients, choosing your food wisely is obviously important. Because you might sacrifice or compromise your nutritional needs, it would be foolish to cut out foods from your diet merely for the sake of cutting down on calories. If you're to win the losing game safely and for any reasonable length of time, you must eat a balanced — but calorie-reduced — diet. I can hear the question already: "But how do I know if I'm consuming a well-balanced diet?" The answer is that you could take several steps to ensure that you're eating properly. One of the easiest and most practical is to simply eat foods selected from each of the following four basic food groups:

The Milk Group (including milk, ice cream, cheese and yogurt)

Most of the body's calcium comes from milk and milk products. Calcium builds bones and teeth and helps the muscles, heart and nerves function properly. Foods in this group also provide the body with significant amounts of protein, riboflavin (Vitamin B2), Vitamin A, and other important nutrients.

The Meat Group (including meat, poultry, fish and eggs)

This group provides the body with protein, which is essential for strength and for maintaining and repairing body tissue. Young people need protein to grow. It also helps form the red blood cells and antibodies you need to fight infection. Foods in this group also provide the body with iron, thiamine (Vitamin B), riboflavin (Vitamin B2), and niacin. Among other sources of protein are peanut butter, lima beans and soybeans.

The Vegetable/Fruit Group

Dark green and yellow vegetables and apples, pears and bananas provide various vitamins, minerals and fiber. Citrus fruits, strawberries, cantaloupe, tomatoes, cabbage, potatoes, green peppers and broccoli provide Vitamin C.

The Bread and Cereal Group

Foods in this group, especially those made from enriched or restored whole grain, provide the body with a large amount of iron, niacin, the B vitamins, and carbohydrates. These high-carbohydrate foods provide energy, and many have significant amounts of fiber, which is also vital for your health.

The recommended daily servings from the four basic food groups outlined above are two servings each from the milk group; two from the meat and protein-rich foods group; four servings from the cereal group; and four from the fruits and vegetables group.

These recommendations are for an average person. Larger and more active people need more servings, as do pregnant and nursing women, and young people in their growth years. If you have variety in your food choices and select from nutrient-dense foods, these servings will of themselves supply essentially all necessary nutrients—no matter how large you are or how actively you exercise.

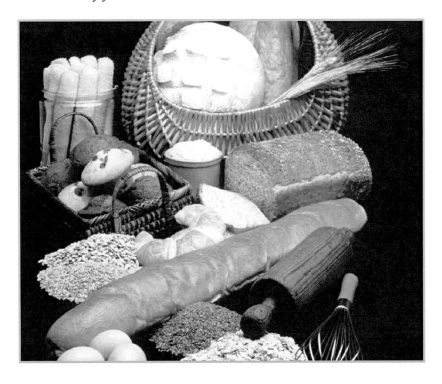

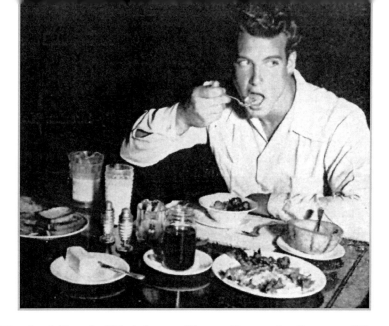

Typical Day's Diet from Steve Reeve's Competition Days

Back when I was competing, a typical day's diet would be perfectly balanced, starting with a special energy drink I always consumed, and that my friend, John Little, has since named, "The Steve Reeves Power Drink." Here's the recipe, along with the rest of my foods for the day and my training schedule, (so you can see how everything fits in).

8:00 a.m. — Breakfast:

The Steve Reeves Power Drink

(prepared in a blender)

14 ounces of freshly squeezed orange juice

1 tablespoon of Knox gelatin

1 tablespoon of honey

1 banana

2-4 raw eggs (today, pasteurized eggs might be safer)

2 tablespoons of High-Protein Powder (I make my own.)

9 a.m. to 11 a.m. — Workout

(On either Monday, Wednesday, or Friday)

Noon — Lunch:

Cottage cheese (with a handful of nuts, raisins)

Two pieces of fresh fruit (in season)

Early evening—Dinner:

One huge salad

One Swordfish steak (or turkey, tuna or lean ground beef)

Hit a Home Run by Making Your Own Protein Powder

You can make your own protein powder by combining:

1/2 lb. of powdered egg whites

1/2 lb. of powdered skim milk

1/4 lb. of powdered soy protein

Cover all your bases by using a combination of animal and vegetable protein. The powdered egg whites put you on first base, nutritionally speaking. The powdered skim milk gets you to second base. The powdered soy protein puts you on third base — and, by adding gelatin to this mixture, you score a home run!

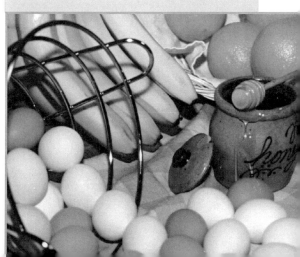

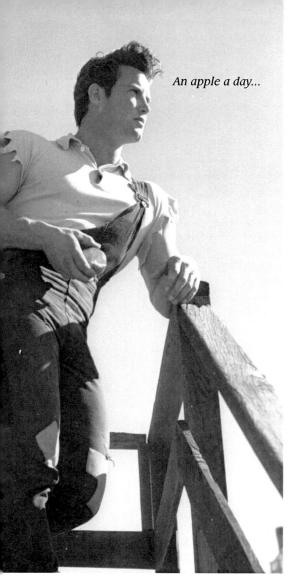

An apple a day...

As you can see, this diet is very well-balanced with something from each of the food groups included. As breakfast is the first meal of the day, it sets your pace — energy wise — for the duration of the day. Another great, high-energy breakfast would be as follows:

> Cut an apple into small cubes.
> Grate a small carrot. Add the following:
> 1/4 cup of raw oatmeal
> 1/4 cup of bran
> 2 teaspoons bee pollen
> 1/4 cup of wheat germ
> 1/4 cup almonds
> 1 heaping tablespoon of honey
> 1 cup milk (I personally prefer goat's milk because it is more complete)

This great breakfast just invigorates you and is tremendous fuel for your Classic Physique workouts! I also recommend that your daily diet consist of 60 percent of calories from complex carbohydrates and natural simple carbs (such as whole fruits), 20 percent from protein and not more than 20 percent from fat. Also, when in serious training, you'll find it advantageous to eat your complex carbohydrates prior to your workout and then, after your workout, consume your protein throughout the rest of the day to help in the process of growth and repair.

It's even advantageous the day before your workout (for example, on Sundays, Tuesdays and Thursdays) to eat predominantly complex carbohydrates starting with lunch, to ensure that your energy levels are amped to the maximum for your workout the next day. For example, you could start out your pre-workout day diet by having oatmeal with a few almonds thrown in, plus apples and raisins for breakfast. You could also eat as many bananas as you wished throughout the course of the day. You might even want to indulge in a little pasta in the form of wholewheat spaghetti with a sauce that didn't have any meat or oil in it. In addition, on these high-carb pre-workout days you could also have some cornbread or cornmeal mush and buckwheat — all foods that are high in complex carbohydrates.

Sometimes even today when I've finished such a high-carb breakfast, lunch and dinner, the next day I'm feeling so great and energetic that I feel like going out and tipping my truck over! I mean, I literally feel like I have that much energy after I've been on my high carbs! Then, on the day that I workout, I'll consume half of my calories from complex carbohydrates and the remainder from protein in order to rebuild what I've torn down from the workout.

Again, keep the diet well-balanced, with a slight emphasis on your complex carbohydrates, and you'll have abundant energy that will last you not only through the most demanding of workouts, but throughout your normal day-to-day activities as well.

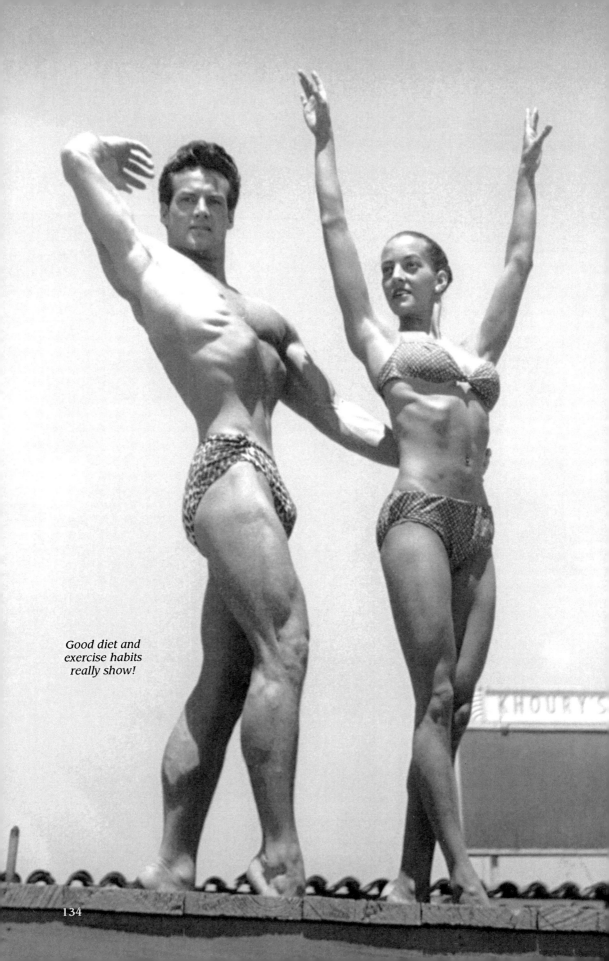

Good diet and exercise habits really show!

Chapter 25: Losing Body Fat

Most people who are starting bodybuilding want to do one of two things: either gain muscle weight or lose body fat. Gaining muscle mass is primarily a matter of training, which has been dealt with successfully elsewhere in this book. This chapter shall attempt to explain to you exactly what you need to know — nutritionally — about losing body fat safely and effectively.

Nothing Magical about Fat Loss

Contrary to what you may have read in most of the muscle magazines, there is nothing "magical" or secretive about losing body fat. I know of many personal trainers who would have you believe that you "must" go to only them for the secret — but there's no such thing. At least, not for anyone who bothers to take the time to actually look into the process of weight loss. The key is a strict adherence to one approach — LOGIC.

Basically, all weight change can be viewed as the end product of a weight-control continuum, which can be envisioned as a teeter-totter; on one end is the food you eat (the energy going into your body), while sitting on the other end is the calories you expend (or the energy going out). If the amount of food you consume (your energy-in) exceeds the amount of your energy used up through activity (your energy-out), the teeter-totter tips to the side of energy-in, and you gain weight. If the amount of food you consume is less than your energy expenditure, then the teeter-totter tips to the side of energy-out and you lose weight. If you want to maintain your present weight, all you have to do is develop an understanding of the factors that affect each end of the teeter-totter and then adopt a "balanced" approach to maintaining this equilibrium.

Most nutritional scientists have advised that the maximum amount of body fat you can lose in any given week is approximately two pounds. Sure, you can lose more weight than that in the course of a week of super-strict dieting, but the chances are that not all of that weight will be fat tissue — in fact, plenty of it will probably be lean muscle tissue! Since there are 3,500 calories in a pound of body fat, this means that if you want to lose two pounds in one week, you'll have to achieve a negative calorie balance at week's end of 7,000 calories (or 3,500 x 2 pounds). In other words, your energy expenditure at the end of the week has to exceed your caloric input by 7,000 calories.

Maintaining a negative calorie balance for the purpose of losing body fat is not a difficult thing to achieve. Just remember the teeter-totter analogy and keep to the side of "more energy-out" rather than "more energy-in." It helps to have an understanding of the caloric value of the various foods you are consuming on a daily basis as well as the amount of calories burned through various activities. And remember, the less body fat that you have in proportion to your lean muscle mass, the easier it is to lose the remaining unwanted fat because it takes more energy to nourish and maintain muscle than it does fat.

I've prepared two charts — one for the caloric values of specific foods and the other for the energy expended by the average man (weighing 150 pounds) in various activities:

Caloric Value of Specific Foods

Food	Weight/Measure	Calories
Milk Group		
Cheese, Cheddar	1-1/8-inch cube	115
Cheese, cottage, creamed	1/4 cup	65
Cream (in coffee)	1 tbsp.	30
Milk, fluid, skim	1 cup	90
Milk, fluid, whole	1 cup	160
Meat Group		
Beans, canned (from dry)	3/4 cup	233
Beef, pot roast	3 oz.	245
Chicken	1/2 breast (with bone)	155
Egg	1 medium	80
Haddock	1 fillet	140
Ham, boiled	2 oz.	135
Hot dog	1 medium	170
Liver, beef	2 oz.	130
Peanut butter	2 tbsp.	190
Pork chop	1 chop	260
Salmon, canned	1/2 cup	120
Sausage, bologna	2 slices	173
Vegetable Group		
Beans, snap, green	1/2 cup	15
Broccoli	1/2 cup	20
Cabbage, shredded, raw	1/2 cup	10
Carrots, diced	1/2 cup	23
Corn, canned	1/2 cup	85
Lettuce leaves	2 large or 4 small	10
Peas, green	1/2 cup	58
Potato, white	1 medium	90
Spinach	1/2 cup	20
Squash, winter	1/2 cup	65
Sweet potato	1 medium	155
Tomato juice, canned	1/2 cup (small glass)	23

Food	Weight/Measure	Calories
Fruit Group		
Apple, raw	1 medium	70
Apricots, dried/stewed	1/2 cup	135
Banana, raw	1 medium	100
Cantaloupe	1/2 melon	60
Grapefruit	1/2 medium	45
Orange	1 medium	65
Orange juice, fresh	1/2 cup (small glass)	55
Peaches, canned	1/2 cup with syrup	100
Pineapple juice, canned	1/2 cup (small glass)	68
Prunes, dried, cooked	5 with juice	160
Strawberries, raw	1/2 cup, capped	30
Bread/Cereal Group		
Bread, white, enriched	1 slice	70
Cornflakes, fortified	1-1/3 cup	133
Macaroni, enriched, cooked	3/4 cup	115
Oatmeal, cooked	2/3 cup	87
Rice, cooked	3/4 cup	140
Fats Group		
Bacon, crisp	2 slices	90
Butter or margarine	1 tbsp.	100
Oils, salad or cooking	1 tbsp.	125
Sweets Group		
Beverages (cola)	6 oz.	75
Sugar, granulated	1 tbsp.	40

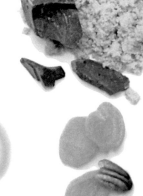

Energy Expended by a 150-Pound Person in Various Activities

To adjust these figures for greater weight than that shown in the reference sample below, simply add 7 percent for each 11 pounds above reference weight, and subtract 7 percent for each 11 pounds below reference weight. This modification will be only approximate, since all of these numbers are only averages.

Activity	Calories Per Hour
Rest and Light Activity	
Lying down or sleeping	80
Sitting	100
Driving a car	120
Standing	140
Moderate Activity	
Bicycling (5-1/2 mph)	210
Walking (2-1/2 mph)	210
Canoeing (2-1/2 mph)	230
Golf	250
Bowling	270
Fencing	300
Rowing (2-1/2 mph)	300
Swimming (1/4 mph)	300
Walking (3-3/4 mph)	300
Badminton	300
Horseback riding (trotting)	350
Volleyball	350
Rollerblading	350
Vigorous Activity	
Table tennis	360
Ice-skating (10 mph)	400
Chopping wood	400
Tennis	420
Water-skiing	480
Hill climbing (100 ft. per hr.)	490
Downhill skiing (10 mph)	600
Squash/handball	600
Cycling (13 mph)	660
Scull rowing (race)	840
Swimming (2 mph)	900
Running (10 mph)	900
Power Walking (5 mph)	900

As you can see by the energy expenditure table, the number of calories you burn can range anywhere from 80 per hour for sleeping to approximately 900 per hour for activities in which most of your body's muscle groups are involved (particularly in Power Walking to which I've devoted an entire chapter elsewhere in this book). As a rule of thumb, the more muscle groups involved in an activity, the greater the energy or caloric expenditure.

Retraining Your Eating Habits

Your eating habits are a major factor in being overweight. In many instances, your habits dictate when and how you eat, what you eat, and how much you eat. Take for example the habit of eating quickly. Your body's mechanism for letting you know when you've had enough to eat is based on your blood-sugar level. The intake of food prompts a relatively slow response on this level. When you eat rapidly, you often eat more food than you normally would before the satiety mechanism has a chance to work. Another example is the practice of eating your meals in front of the television set and developing a habit of eating something every time you watch television, regardless of whether or not it's meal time. And if you're a person who has a cup of coffee and a dessert every time a neighbor drops in for a chat, you've developed a bad habit as far as weight control is concerned.

The key to fat loss is to eat three normal meals a day and, if at all possible, avoid snacking in between meals. Change your living patterns that contribute to snacking and other bad eating habits. Keep a record of what you eat and when you eat it. Many people snack unconsciously. Every time you eat something, think of it as making a deposit in your body's energy bank and remember that too many deposits will result in unwanted fat gain. Never eat after 6:00 p.m. or three hours prior to going to bed.

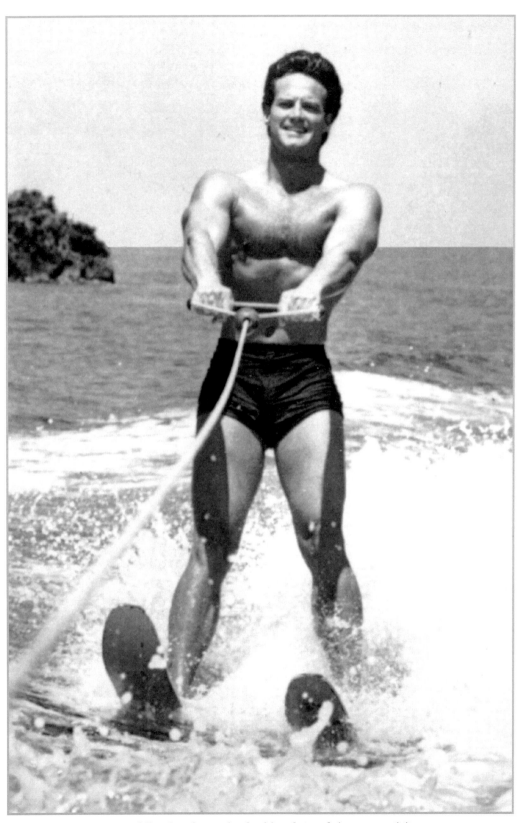
Water-skiing is a fun and refreshing form of vigorous activity.

Chapter 26: Rules to Live By

When I was in the Army and stationed in Japan during 1946, I kept a little black book of health and hygiene tips that I found both true and effective in cultivating outstanding health and fitness habits. I would like to share these "rules to live by" with you now:

1. Drink a glass of warm water with lemon and honey before breakfast.

2. Take a cold shower each morning upon arising — let the cold water run on your genitals for a minute or two to stimulate circulation — then dry off by rubbing briskly with a good Turkish towel.

3. Brush your teeth four times a day: once after each meal, and once before going to bed.

4. Eat a balanced diet of good wholesome food. Eliminate the use of white flour products, white sugar and watch your salt intake.

5. Make your meals pleasant: Eat food you enjoy and chew it well.

6. Drink eight to 12 glasses of water daily.

7. Wash your face daily with warm water, a washcloth and soap. Rinse with cold water.

8. Your skin should be scrubbed briskly with a brush or a loofah once a week. After this treatment, oil should be rubbed into the skin.

9. Brush your hair and massage your scalp daily. If your scalp is dry, rub hot olive oil on your scalp before shampooing.

10. Your body should be exposed to the fresh air and sunlight for one hour a day when the weather permits. Be sure to use a good sunblock (I use one with aloe vera).

11. Form the habit of elimination at least once daily, preferably in the morning before working out or going to work.

12. Keep a tranquil mind and positive attitude at all times; and make your exercise periods a pleasure, not drudgery.

13. Train three times a week and drink lemon and honey in water, prior to your workouts for energy.

14. Get plenty of sleep and rest. Sleep on a fairly hard bed, on your back, with a window open for fresh air.

15. Walk tall and maintain good posture at all times.

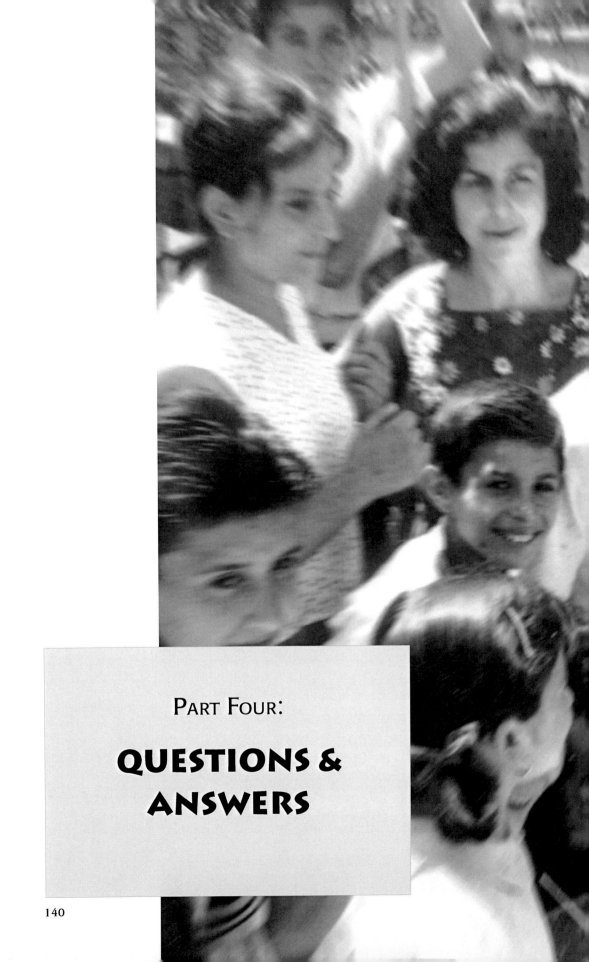

Part Four:

QUESTIONS & ANSWERS

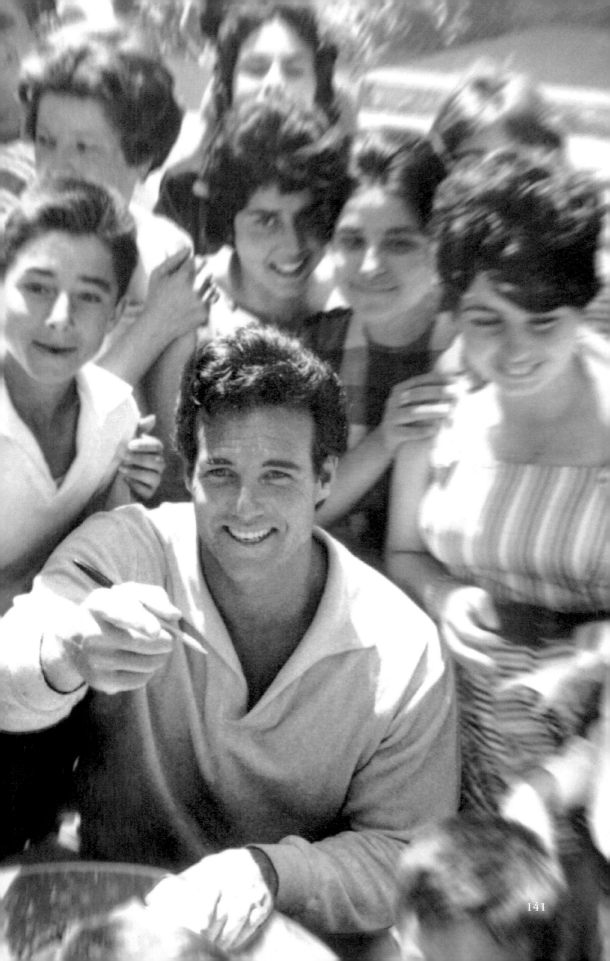

Chapter 27:
A Bodybuilding Seminar with Steve Reeves

Steve Reeves and John Little talk at length on the many aspects of bodybuilding training, nutrition and the lifestye.

The Role of Supplements

QUESTION: Steve, you've stressed the need for a well-balanced diet, but everywhere these days you keep hearing about "supplements." Did you ever take any food supplements when you were building your Classic Physique?

STEVE REEVES: Well I would take products such as Knox Gelatin and Brewer's Yeast. The interesting thing about the gelatin is that it's about 87-percent protein but your body can't utilize the protein efficiently because it's missing two key amino acids which you'll find in eggs. So, if you want to do like I did, and use gelatin as the source of your protein, then make sure that you have eggs with it or else it won't work for you.

There's a wonderful anabolic and health promoting component to gelatin — or at least I found that to be the case. I recall some years ago that I was diagnosed with a duodenal ulcer. I'm not big on hospitals, so their advice to me was to stay home — in bed — and follow a bland diet. I'm a very intuitive individual and I think my intuition cured me of the ulcer — and here's how: I had this incredible craving for Jell-O. I would eat bowls of the stuff during this period and I would thicken it with plain gelatin every day.

Within two months, the symptoms of the duodenal ulcer had disappeared. And when I went back for an X-ray the doctors told me that not only was I completely cured, but there was no sign of scar tissue, either.

I believe to this day that the pure protein within the gelatin helped to cure me. Anyway, you can buy gelatin in any grocery store or health food store. It's about 87-percent protein, as mentioned — but make sure you eat eggs with it or else you won't develop as fast.

More on the "Steve Reeves Power Drink"

QUESTION: For the bodybuilders who, after reading this book, want to try your bodybuilding and nutritional programs, how should they go about mixing up the gelatin and when should they take it?

STEVE REEVES: First off, they needn't take this exclusively. I mean they can get their protein from sources such as tuna, chicken, turkey or even really lean beef. However, if they wanted to try the "Steve Reeves Power Drink," they should make sure that they have at least one egg — separate from the drink if they prefer (in which case it should be soft boiled

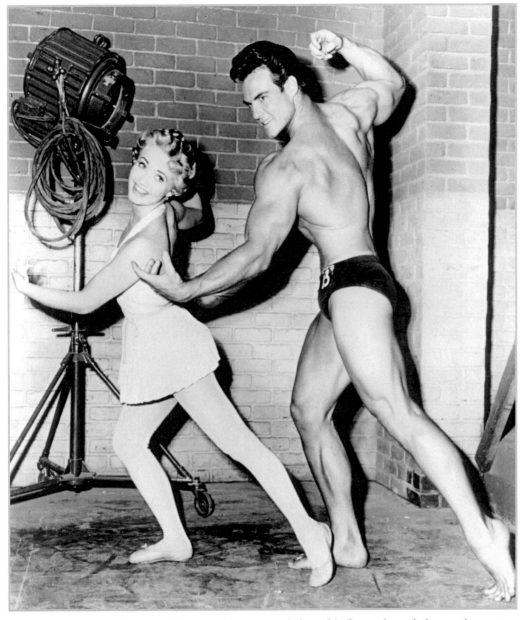
Steve, always willing to introduce his sport and share his fitness knowledge, assists costar Jane Powell in a mock posing routine while on the set of "Athena" (1954).

---

or poached. If it must be fried, they should fry it until it just barely turns white) or mixed in with the gelatin and orange juice mixture I mentioned in the previous chapter.

A Special Workout Electrolyte Replacement Drink

QUESTION: What about replacing the electrolytes that you use up in perspiration during a hard workout? How do you replenish them?

STEVE REEVES: Well, interestingly enough, I automatically did something to redress this balance when I was working out heavily years ago. I didn't know of it's biochemical properties at the time, of course, but I knew instinctively that my body required the ingredients I put into a special drink that I would sip on during my workouts. Now, they call this "electrolyte replacement" drinks such as Gatorade and the like.

But I used to drink a lot of water and I used to mix lemon and honey with my water and that was how I was able to replace all of my electrolytes that were lost through perspiration — and it worked great. Something instinctively told me that these nutrients were needed by my body during a workout in order to continue working out at optimum levels.

By having the lemon juice and honey, I was able to maintain my body's acid balance, and I had more energy and was able to get much more work out of my muscles without tiring them too prematurely. In other words, my muscles would tire out due to genuine muscle fatigue as opposed to some biochemical imbalance.

> **THE STEVE REEVES ELECTROLYTE WORKOUT FORMULA**
>
> *(To be consumed during your workouts)*
>
> Mix the following together:
>
> 1/2-cup lemon juice
>
> 3-tablespoonsful of honey (mix thoroughly until the lemon juice dissolves the honey)
>
> Then mix in with a half-gallon of water. Consume the entire half gallon during your workout by taking two to three sips after each set.

The Importance of Water

QUESTION: You mentioned the importance of consuming water in your chapter on nutrition and you've mentioned that one should drink about a half gallon of it during one's workout. Why is water so important for the bodybuilder?

STEVE REEVES: It is very important to drink a lot of water while you exercise. I've touched on the importance of water in the chapter on nutrition, but let me elaborate on its significance to the bodybuilder. First off, more than 75 percent of your muscles are composed of water. Secondly, water serves to help the bodybuilder metabolize body fat. In other words, when you workout, if you don't have sufficient water intake, you're going to be burning glycogen exclusively and you'll run out of energy far too soon for your workout to be as productive as it should be. If you can get your body to burn fat, as well as glycogen, you won't burn out as quickly and you'll have a leaner physique as well. Water really helps you to burn fat and build your muscles, so don't scrimp on consuming it throughout the day.

Building vs. Bulking

QUESTION: How many calories would you consume to build up when, for instance, you were in a bulking stage?

STEVE REEVES: I never was in a bulking stage, preferring to be in a building stage. When I'm saying is that a lot of people would in fact bulk up, then trim down for shows, contests, pictures, whatever — but every pound of muscle that I put on was good muscle, all throughout my career.

I first started serious bodybuilding when I was 16 years old and I joined Yarick's Gym weighing 163 pounds. I worked out for a month, and I got on the scale looking a little better; more firmed up, more in shape — but I still weighed 163 pounds. But that month served to tone up my body and get my metabolism working properly for gaining muscle.

Then the following month I got on the scale and weighed 173 pounds — I had gained 10 pounds of solid muscle! You could actually see it growing! The next month brought another

10 pounds. In one more month, I gained 10 more pounds. After working out at Yarick's Gym for only four months, I gained 30 pounds of solid muscle — going from 163 to 193 pounds!

Guys who had been working out for three and four years before me couldn't believe it! They thought a miracle had happened there. But never did I simply try to gain weight or fat in an effort to look bigger or "bulk" up. It was quality muscle all the way or I didn't want it.

Do Not Impose Limitations on your Development

QUESTION: What do you think accounted for your rapid muscular progress?

STEVE REEVES: I think, number one, because I didn't know it was difficult to build muscles. Nobody told me, "Boy, that's really hard or impossible to achieve." Or, "You have to work for years before you can gain an inch on your arms." It's not that I was different than any of you reading this book — but I refused to accept limitations on what I could achieve with my bodybuilding.

I also used extreme concentration. When I worked out, I'd concentrate exclusively on the muscle I was training. I'd concentrate on the movements and perform them nice and slow so that I could really feel the movement all the way up and all the way down. I used a full range of motion and it really worked out well for me. You have to establish a superior line of communication between your brain and your muscles, and you can only do that two ways: by concentration and by practicing muscle-control exercises in your spare time when you're not working out.

When you can flip those muscles — that is, getting them to flex or twitch through brief, voluntary contraction, you know you have great communication between your mind and your muscle tissue. So, by building up a greater, superior line of communication between my brain and my muscles, I was able to develop much faster and easier than most of my contemporaries.

I didn't put so much time into my training, either. I'd workout only three days a week for about 2 or 2-1/2 hours a workout. The other four days a week I would rest because rest is just as important as the workout itself for building muscle size. A lot of bodybuilders don't have adequate recuperation in between workouts. They workout, then they workout, and then they workout again — they're tearing down muscles and not giving them enough rest for optimum growth.

Steve's All Time Best Condition

QUESTION: Looking back now, what did you consider to have been your all-time best condition?

STEVE REEVES: I'd have to say the Mr. America contest because I had a lot of time to prepare for it. I had six months to prepare for that contest. I got out of the Army in October of 1946. I was 20 years old and worked out for two months and won my first contest in December of 1946 (Mr. Pacific Coast in Portland, Oregon). And then I had from January all the way through the middle of June to prepare for the contest, so that was my best shape then. I was peaking, peaking, peaking.

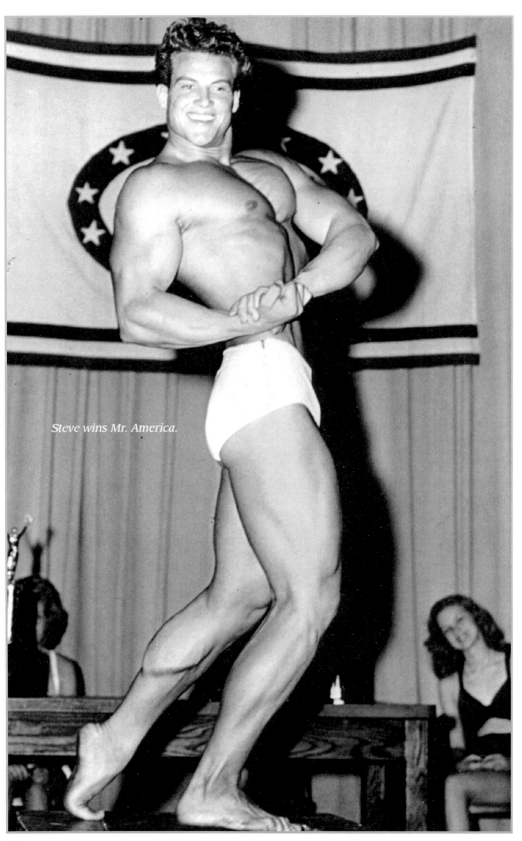

Steve wins Mr. America.

After that contest I went to acting school and, from then on, just worked out to maintain myself. Then, I'd get discouraged if somebody said, "Well, you're not doing so well in your movie career." Or, "You haven't even got your career started yet. Why don't you workout again and become Mr. Universe?" So in despair, I'd work out for three weeks and win a contest. I found that I could always get back within about a month any muscle I may have lost.

TRAINING FOR FILMS

QUESTION: How long did you have to train to prepare for your many film roles?

STEVE REEVES: Probably nowhere near as long as you might think. I only needed about one solid month of training to get back into top shape. In fact, during one period when I was busy making movies, I only worked out one month a year — which was usually April. I didn't have many weights, I think I had a pair of 50-pound dumbbells that were adjustable.

At this point I was living in Switzerland and had a boxer dog and during the winter I would hike through the woods for a couple hours a day. When I did the movies, all the Swiss food made me about 10 pounds overweight. So I would workout for about a month, increasing my walks from two hours to three and working out with the weights at the gym. I also went on a low-fat diet. I'd end up in good shape. And during the filming, I would sweat so much that I'd never gain any fat anyway. So, with the help of good nutrition, the muscle I built up would stay with me for up to nine months afterwards.

TOP FORM MEASUREMENTS

QUESTION: In order to set the record straight once and for all, what were your measurements when you were in your all-time top shape?

STEVE REEVES: My best measurements were as follows:

Height: 6-foot-1-inch
Weight: 215 pounds
Shoulder breadth: 23-1/2 inches
Neck: 18-1/4 inches
Chest: 52 inches
Waist: 29 inches
Hips: 38 inches
Biceps: 18-1/4 inches
Forearms: 14-3/4 inches
Wrist: 7-1/4 inches
Thigh: 26 inches
Calf: 18-1/4 inches
Ankle: 9-1/4 inches

BALANCING YOUR PROPORTIONS

QUESTION: Were your arms always in proportion to your neck and calves?

STEVE REEVES: No, it's funny that when I started working out at Yarick's Gym, my arms were only 13-1/2-inches, but my calves were 16-inches, which made them two-and-a-half inches out of proportion initially. In an attempt to keep my body balanced, I didn't work my

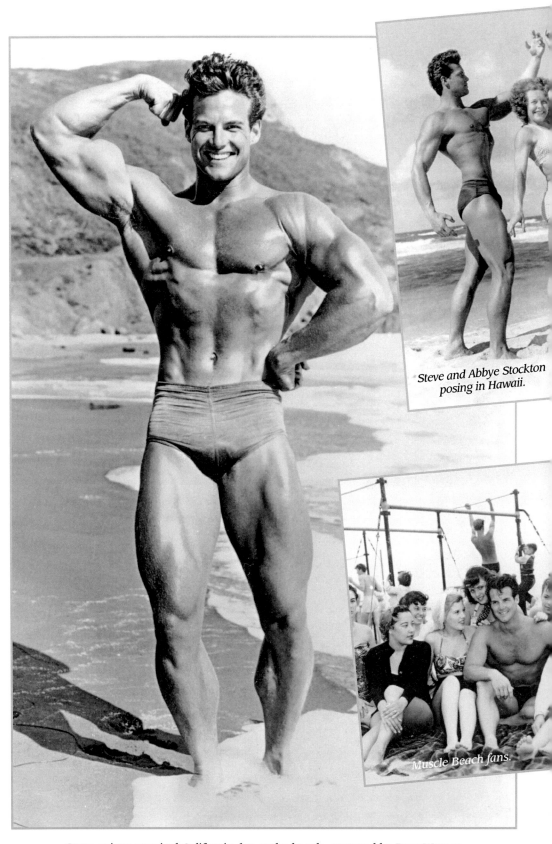

Steve and Abbye Stockton posing in Hawaii.

Muscle Beach fans.

Steve enjoys a typical California day at the beach, captured by Russ Warner.

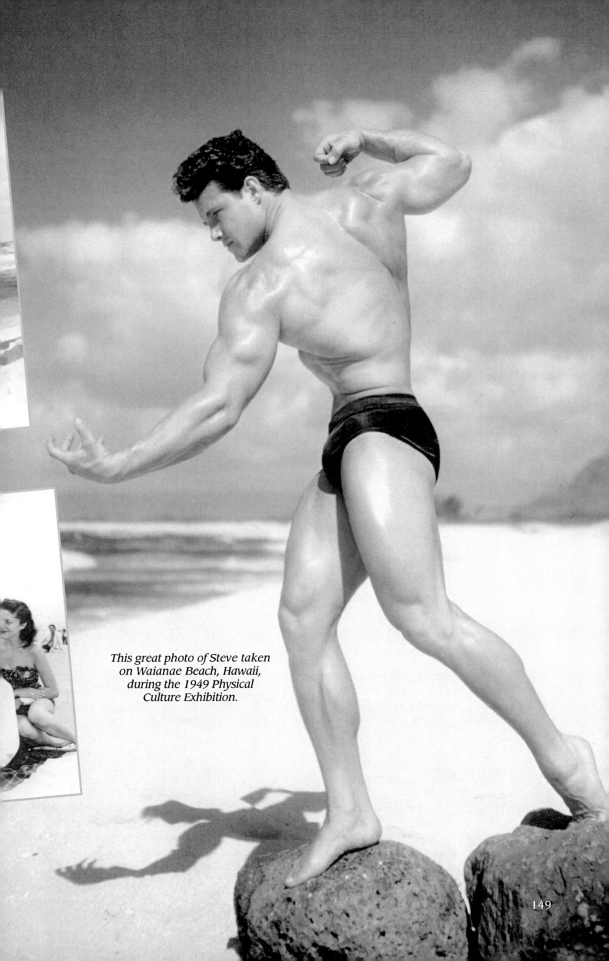

This great photo of Steve taken on Waianae Beach, Hawaii, during the 1949 Physical Culture Exhibition.

calves at all until I brought my arms up to 16-inches. And then I built my arms, my neck and my calves up to 17-inches together; 17-1/2 inches together; 18-inches together; 18-1/2 inches together, and I left them at that. That was plenty for me.

More on Taking Measurements

QUESTION: Were these measurements you've just listed taken "cold," — that is, a natural measurement, unaffected by pumping the muscle up prior to taping it?

STEVE REEVES: Yes, that's exactly how they were taken. Many bodybuilders today give measurements after they are pumped up. When I was training hard, we would take our measurements when we got up in the morning — before we exercised. We never measured ourselves after exercising or after having just pumped up or anything like that. Our measurements were always taken cold — I mean, ice cold. And we would have other guys take the measurements for us to ensure that they were accurately recorded. I'd measure George Eiferman's arm, Armand Tanny would measure my arm — it didn't matter. I mean, we knew what we had, we weren't trying to con anybody. And we knew it was going to be the same measurement the next day because we knew that what we had was not there because of steroids, which we didn't take, but because of training, and therefore, it wasn't going to disappear if we stopped taking such things. I mean, these guys today, if they don't take their steroids, a week later their arms shrink by inches.

THOUGHTS ON "MODERN" TRAINING METHODS

QUESTION: Speaking of the guys today, what are your thoughts regarding the routines advocated by today's champions — the six days per week, 20 sets per body part routines?

STEVE REEVES: I think it's ridiculous and a waste of time! I think those who engage in such training would get twice as much benefit — with half as much work — and much more pleasure out of training my way. Here's how I look at it: On my system, when you're working your muscle groups, you're also working your nervous system with the concentration and stress of trying to get those last reps in only three sets. With such a compact degree of work, you don't think about all those other sets that are coming up next, with the result that you can really put out a maximal effort. And then you have days off and your body is able to recuperate and get even stronger than it was before.

But if you're going to exercise twice a day, six times a week, when do you have time to recuperate? You don't! And if you're going to do so many exercises and so many sets, you can't be giving your all to your workout because it wouldn't be possible. You just couldn't. It's just like jogging compared to running. I believe in running. In fact, I used to run the mile just for exercise years ago and I always tried to complete it within five minutes. I used to do that about twice a week. The world record wasn't even four minutes at that time. I worked up to that, too. I paced myself. In any event, the point is this: When people jog, they have to hold back. If they were going to run a marathon, for instance, they would have to hold themselves back from what they were fully capable of — in terms of their all-out sprinting capacity — because if they were giving their all, they would be out of wind at about 200 yards!

The same thing applies for people who train twice a day, six days a week. They can't be giving their all to their workout because it's impossible to give maximum effort that many times a day, that many days per week, without getting stale and starting to hate your workouts instead of enjoying them.

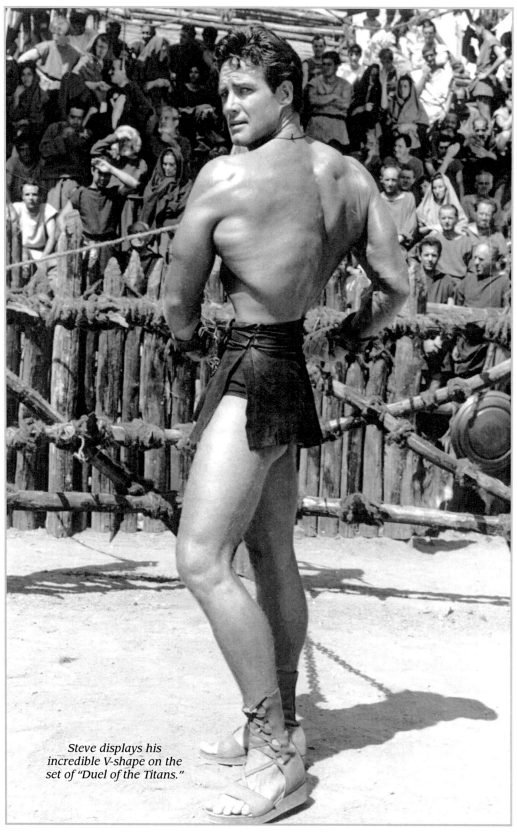

Steve displays his incredible V-shape on the set of "Duel of the Titans."

I Never Felt Overtrained on the "Classic Physique" Schedule

QUESTION: Did you ever find that performing nine sets per body part, two and one-half hours per workout, three times per week, such as you recommend in your Classic Physique schedule, left you feeling overtrained or tired?

STEVE REEVES: Never. The reason is that I got a total of four days rest each week. In other words, I was training maybe seven hours a week — total time — and that was it. There are 168 hours in a week, so I never felt overtrained, never. In fact, I never had to take layoffs from training or anything like that because I never felt overtrained. I would always go into a workout looking forward to it; seeing if I could do a few more reps that day, or maybe raise the weight a little bit. I always felt recharged and ready for my next workout.

A Novel Leg Training Discovery

QUESTION: You mentioned earlier that you learned which exercises affected different muscles the best by testing them out on yourself when you were stationed in the Philippines during World War II, and then seeing where you felt the soreness the next day. Were there any other "discoveries" you made during that period?

STEVE REEVES: Yes, in fact it was during that period that I discovered an exercise that is really difficult to do — and that produces terrific results for the legs. Put half of your body weight on a bar and squat 100 times with it. I am referring to a full squat, by the way, so that the backs of your thighs touch your calves. Do this for 100 repetitions in a row without pause. If you do it too fast, you'll find that you play out; your muscles will get too shaky and weak. But if you do it too slow, that bar on your back is going to kill you. You have to time it exactly right. The reason that I did this was that, being in the Army (I was stationed in the Philippines and in Japan), I only had 100 pounds to start with, and 100 pounds just isn't enough to do squats with — unless you did a lot of them. So I started with 50 reps and the next week I went up to 55. Then the following week, I went up to 60 reps until I eventually got to where I could squat with it 100 times. It's a really demanding exercise. It also improved my cardiovascular conditioning a lot in the process, and my legs kept in great shape! My weight at the time was around 200 pounds, so that 100 pounds was exactly half my bodyweight. If a fellow weighs 300 pounds, then he would use 150 pounds.

I told a lot of fellows about this workout and they wouldn't do it. Bodybuilders today with their huge thighs won't do it! They don't want to take the chance of not being able to complete it. But try it out for yourself and see if your legs don't respond — and quickly!

Gee, Your Triceps Look "Swell"

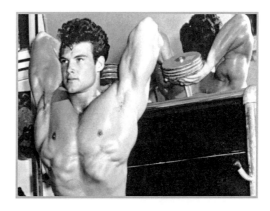

QUESTION: Your triceps look incredible — not to mention your other body parts — particularly the lateral head. Your triceps development, being so many years ahead of everybody else's, must have drawn a lot of attention. Do you recall any of the reactions that people had to your arms?

STEVE REEVES: Your question reminds me of a funny story. When I was going into the Army, we had to get shots. Most soldiers would get a shot of some sort to immunize them when they were in the service. And I recall going in to get my needle and when I came out of the doctor's office, there was a fellow waiting in line who looked really nervous. As I came out he asked, "How was it, man? Was it really bad?"

And I said "No, I don't think so — my arm's not swollen too much." And I rolled up my sleeve and flexed the lateral head of my triceps hard so that it bulged out as far as it could. That poor fellow's face went green!

The Incline Dumbbell Curl — the "Perfect" Biceps Exercise

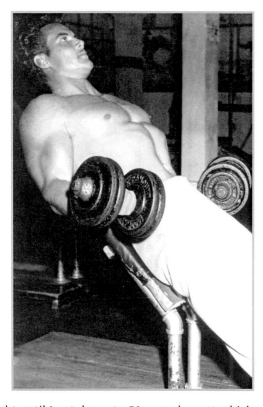

QUESTION: You mentioned in the chapter, "Building the Classic Physique," that you recommend three different biceps exercises to be performed for three sets each. Yet didn't you eventually use only one exercise — the incline curl — for your biceps? Why isn't this the movement you recommend in this chapter for developing your biceps?

STEVE REEVES: Simply because the incline curl was not the only movement I used to build my biceps. You'll notice, however, that the incline curl was one of the three exercises I listed in the biceps workout — just not at the exclusion of all other exercises. However, if you really want to specialize on your biceps for an upcoming contest or event, and you find — as I did — that the incline curl really does the job for you, then you should utilize it in the same fashion that I did: I would start out the incline curl with 75 pounds for 7 reps (I could strict curl 90-pound dumbbells — but only for one rep). On my next set, I would reduce the weight to 70 pounds. And then with each succeeding set, I would reduce the weight until I got down to 50 pounds — at which I would remain for the duration of my sets. I wouldn't let myself drop the weight below 50 pounds, and I would perform 9 sets in total of this one movement.

More on Offset Flyes for Chest Development

QUESTION: In your "Building the Classic Physique" routine, you mention using an offset grip when performing dumbbell flyes. I'm still a little unsure as to what this means. Can you elaborate on this technique, please?

STEVE REEVES: Sure. Proper dumbbell flyes should be performed with the thumbs in. Thumbs in with your arms bent to, approximately, a 30-degree angle. It really makes a difference in building up your chest. When your arms are extended above your chest to begin the movement, your palms should be facing your feet so that your thumbs are side by side. Your grip should be off-center so that your thumb and index finger are touching the plates at the top of the dumbbell. I also recommend an offset dumbbell if you can assemble one. In other words, put the plates, jammed against your thumb and have the remainder or lower part of the dumbbell hanging down towards the ground, thereby providing resistance throughout a greater range of motion.

Typical dumbbell flyes — like close-grip bench presses — start out difficult and then get progressively easier towards the top or finish of the movement. This means that there is an imbalance in the resistance. But when flyes are performed my way, with the thumbs in, the resistance is constant and difficult all the way up. I call them offset flyes. And it's important that your elbows be bent to a 30-degree angle, and that you keep your arms bent in this position throughout the entire duration of your set. If I were to tell someone how to do the exercise, I'd tell them to do it as if their arms were in a cast at about a 30-degree angle, and then keep that degree of angle all the way throughout the movement. And offset your plates. In fact, if I really wanted to get a good workout, I'd put two or three plates on the inside and about five on the outside to keep a real angle of resistance on my pecs via an offset grip.

Heavy Weights Are Not the Answer

QUESTION: You keep hitting home the point that good form is so important for building a classic physique — but aren't heavy weights the real answer for building muscle size?

STEVE REEVES: I believe that if you use too much weight before you're ready, it's not good for building muscle size. With heavy weights, your tendons get extra strong but then they tend to take over — instead of the muscle! Whereas if you use the proper weight and do the exercises slowly and with good concentration, the muscles will take over and will build and strengthen.

If you do jerky movements, with too heavy a weight, the tendons are going to get the size of your thumb but your muscles will be slow to gain size! This is not just a theory of mine but it's something I've observed in a great many people who trained in such a fashion over a period of some 50 years. Perfect form with as heavy a weight as you can handle — while still maintaining perfect form — is the key to building a Classic Physique.

You Don't Need Aerobics to Become Defined

QUESTION: When you were training for your Mr. America and Mr. Universe wins, did you ever include any aerobic training along with your bodybuilding workouts in order to become more defined?

STEVE REEVES: No, I never had to. I was always in fairly good shape all year around. If there was a contest coming up, I would simply train a little harder. In other words, I would just train a little bit faster and increase the intensity of my workouts by having less rest time in between sets and muscle groups.

The whole key to acquiring a Classic Physique lies in the proper balance of intensity, duration and frequency of your workouts. If you work out at too high an intensity, you can't work out very long — which means you may stimulate some muscle growth but you'll not burn off much body fat. If, on the other hand, you train with an intensity that is too low, you can go on for long duration — and burn some body fat — but it's too low an intensity to stimulate much increase in muscle size. Training to either extreme is not desirable. It's a waste of time unless you have a balance of both intensity and duration in your workouts, as well as adequate rest periods in between workouts to enhance your recuperation from training.

Finding that "Sweet Spot"

QUESTION: How does one find the ideal balance between intensity and duration in order to insure maximal results from your schedule?

STEVE REEVES: I guess that each individual is different and probably a person with fast-twitch muscle fibers would be best advised to keep his repetitions low; say from five to seven. That would best suit his predominant fiber type. However, a person with slow-twitch muscle fibers could do something with more endurance, such as 12 to 15 reps because he can maintain his efforts for a longer period of time without getting tired. You have to go along with what fiber type you are, but you can modify it slightly.

Proper Rep Speed

QUESTION: What is a good rep speed or cadence to employ for maximum results?

STEVE REEVES: I've always found a good cadence to be three seconds down and two seconds up.

Breathing During Exercise

Question: What about breathing during exercise? Is there an ideal way to breath during training?

Steve Reeves: A lot of people nowadays have a theory that you "blow the weight away from you" when you're training. That is, when you press, for example, a barbell overhead, this pushing motion should be accompanied by a strong exhalation.

Other people are of the opinion — like I am — that you should take a breath in — or hold the breath in — during the point of greatest exertion.

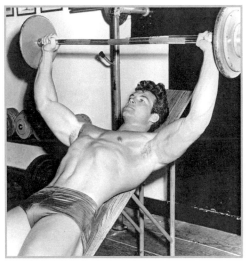

For example, on a bench press, breath in deeply when you lower the bar, before you press it up. The midway point on the way up is the hardest, and you should hold your breath until you pass through the half way point. Some people are afraid of blacking out when they do this because they think they'll hold their breath too long — that won't happen. If you know you're not going to make your rep, then breathe out.

It's very simple. I breathe in just before the positive portion of the rep, and hold it half way through the positive and then let it out during the negative.

The Number One Training Mistake

Question: As not only the greatest bodybuilder in history, but also one of its most dedicated teachers, what is the most common training mistake you've seen repeated in gyms over the years?

Steve Reeves: Without question, it would have to be cheating on an exercise. Using full body swings, instead of just using the muscle groups in isolation, such as the biceps and triceps. Or people bouncing when doing squats or bouncing the weight off their chest when performing bench presses — there's all kinds of cheating.

The only person you cheat when you break good form to handle heavier weight is yourself, because you're robbing your muscles of stimulation they could be using to grow bigger and stronger.

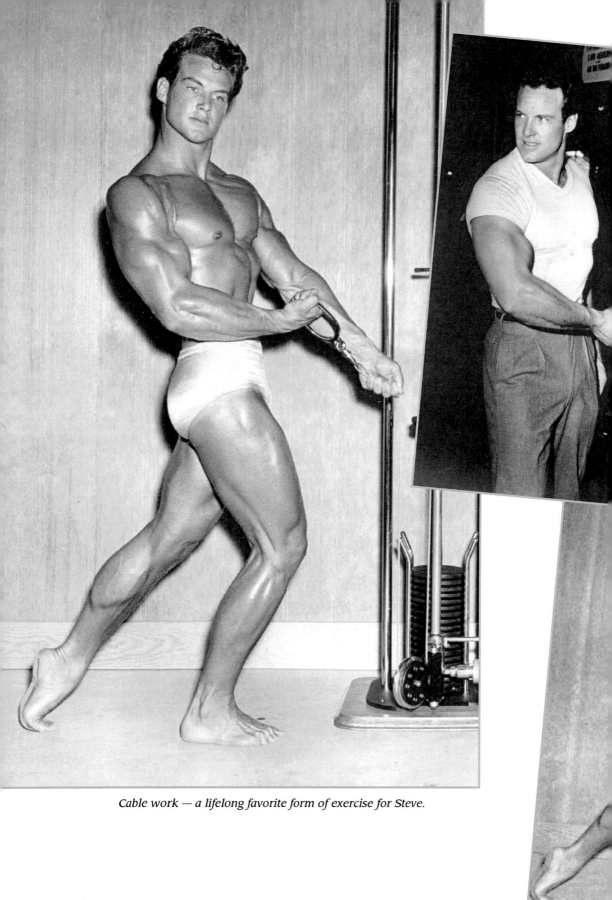

Cable work — a lifelong favorite form of exercise for Steve.

Steve Reeves — Athlete Extraordinaire!

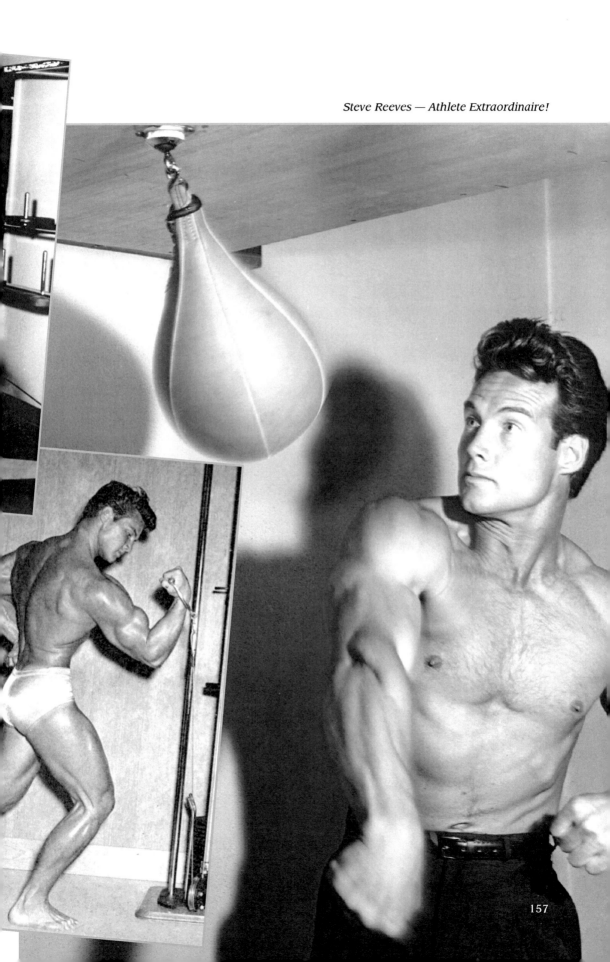

Don't Use a Thumbless Grip

Question: I've seen some guys at my gym using a thumbless grip on their bench presses. What do you think of this practice?

Steve Reeves: I don't believe in it at all. You're not going to get that much more weight doing your presses in such a fashion. For those who are unfamiliar with the term "thumbless grip," it simply means that you move your thumb to the same side of the bar as your fingers, and it's actually a very dangerous thing to do. I knew a man who broke his sternum doing that when the bar rolled out of his hands during a set of bench presses. I always keep my thumb on the opposite side of the bar from my fingers when I'm bench pressing. It's safer — and more productive — that way.

"Rear-Stop Bars" — and How to Make Them

Question: I'd like to know more about the "rear-stop bar" you mentioned in Chapter 14. How would you make it?

Steve Reeves: It's really quite simple. I would make brackets and bolt them onto the back of an incline bench. Then I would get a one-inch bar that will fit through the brackets on the back of the bench. The bar can be about 18 inches to 24 inches long — depending on your shoulder width — and then I'd get some sleeves that I had made out of aluminum. They should be about three inches in diameter so that you don't have all of the pressure of your arm against the stop-bar in one place on your triceps. If it's a three-inch bar — or padded — you won't feel any discomfort, as it's dispersed and not concentrated. This bar, attached to the rear of your incline bench, serves simply to hold your arms in place throughout the performance of incline curls. I think you'll find it as terrific as I did — it really works wonders.

The Reason You Should Train Three Days a Week

Question: Your routine has me in the gym only three days a week. Why do you recommend such a short amount of training time when most champions I read about today are spending up to six days a week in the gym?

Steve Reeves: Well, don't forget that most of the "champions" you read about today are full of anabolic steroids and other such growth-enhancing drugs which make their training programs useless to the natural bodybuilder — which is the only type of bodybuilding I care about. And to this end, when people go to the gym, they should try to maximize their benefit and minimize their time. If they're going to put in two hours, then they should get two hours worth of growth stimulation.

Now, growth stimulation and growth production are two entirely separate animals. When you stimulate growth in the gym, that's only half of the equation. The second half involves recovery and growth — and that only happens when you're at rest. This means that you — obviously— can't be training every day. You need rest in between, otherwise your nerves will get shattered and you lose your enthusiasm. So you need to find the maximum workout you can take, with the ideal amount of recuperation time in between workouts.

It's better to underdo a workout than to overdo a workout. If you overdo your training, then you tear down too much of your recuperative ability and tissue and it defeats your purpose. You have to be aware of that delicate balance that exists so that you don't overtrain.

You should approach each workout full of enthusiasm, not saying, "Oh gee, it's Wednesday,

I guess I've got to go down to the gym." You should look forward to it! You should be saying, "Well, last week I did my inclines with 105-pound dumbbells for eight reps — this time I'm going to try and do it for nine or 10 reps!" Head for the gym each time with a goal firmly fixed in your mind and don't forget to keep charts of your progress from one workout to the next — that is a great source of motivation and shows you what you need to surpass in your next workout!

The "Perfect" Workout Schedule

Question: How would you create the "perfect" workout schedule?

Steve Reeves: I'm of the opinion that the "perfect" workout would see a person work out with a day and a half rest in between sessions. For example, you would workout on Monday morning, Wednesday evening and Saturday morning. That would be a great workout because you would know that you've got a day and a half until you had to hit it again — and you could really put out. I think that would be the perfect workout. In fact, I did try such a schedule when I had my own gym in Miami Beach and it worked out great for me. I had my best measurements at that time: 18-1/4 inch calf, 18-1/4 inch neck and 18-1/4 inch biceps. As I owned the gym, I could workout whenever I wanted to. I only did this for a period of about three months but I got really good results from it — and by "results" I mean on top of the results I already had.

Insert: Steve's biceps — what size and shape — drug free!
Below: The only photo known to exist of Steve in front of his Athletic CLub.

Ideal Rest Time between Sets

Question: When training your various muscle groups, how much rest would you recommend one take in between sets?

Steve Reeves: I'd recommend that the trainee take just enough rest to let your training partner do his set. When I was training, I found that having one training partner was best. If I had two training partners, I'd cool down too much waiting for my turn again, so one training partner is ideal. Take just enough time in between each set for your partner to grab the apparatus and hit it. In other words, use high intensity. By the way, if you don't have a workout partner, figure out how long it takes you to do the set, and rest about the same length of time only. However, in between body parts you can rest up to five minutes.

Keeping the Weight the Same

Question: When training in this fashion, would you increase the weight each set — or would it remain the same?

Steve Reeves: The weight would either remain the same or be reduced slightly — depending on your personal energy levels. You would always try to keep the weight the same and go to your limit on each set for as many reps as you can. It's possible, say, on the first set, that you might hit 12 reps; but you might have to go down to eight reps on the third set because — if you give each set your all — you're not going to be able to recuperate that fast — especially if you just go one after the other with your workout partner.

The Ideal Number of Repetitions

Question: How many repetitions are necessary to fully stimulate a muscle?

Steve Reeves: Oh, I used to do between eight and 12. I figured that was the ideal amount. But sometimes I would mix things up. For instance, I don't believe in keeping the same routine all of the time. In fact, I don't even like to call a workout a "routine." I prefer to call it a "schedule." A routine means doing the same thing over and over and over again. What I like to do is change my schedules. For example, I may use the same exercises, but maybe one day a week, I might do between five and seven repetitions for a muscle group. Another day during the week, I'll do between eight and 12 repetitions for that same muscle group, and on another day I'll shoot for a rep range between 12 and 15. That way you confuse the muscles you're training. The body's used to really exerting for those seven reps when, all of a sudden, you hit it with 15 reps, and it has to change completely. It really works out well.

Monthly Repetition Alternations — A Practical Example

Question: How would a person incorporate this alternating repetition scheme into their training schedule?

Steve Reeves: A person can do it this way: workout one month with five to seven reps, then jump to 11 to 15, and then go somewhere in the middle again. Back and forth each month, instead of changing each week — which is difficult because you have to remember, "How much weight did I use when I did seven reps on the incline bench curl?" You would have to remember three different schedules, you see, with all those different weights and reps, which is difficult for some people unless they keep a training log book. But I believe in mixing it up to kind of confuse the body, so that it doesn't get into a routine and stay there.

Higher Reps for Calves and Abs

Question: Were your repetitions different for, say, your lower body muscles than for your upper body muscles — or were all of your sets done for eight to 12 repetitions?

Steve Reeves: For the most part, my reps stayed in the eight to 12 range, with the exception of abs and calves which were hit for 20 to 25 reps. For example, if I planned on performing 20 reps for my calves, I would select a weight that would allow me to get 20 full reps. I wouldn't use a resistance that would only allow me to get 10 reps, and I wouldn't cheat on my reps. I'd go all the way up and all the way down.

A Calf Training Tip

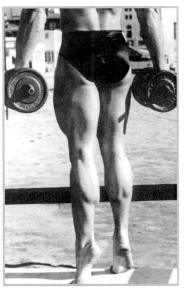

Question: Since you brought up the subject of calf training — and since your calves are so outstanding — do you have any tips you can pass on to us "lesser mortals" who wish to build up our calves?

Steve Reeves: One thing I've found to be highly effective in building the calves is to employ a full range of motion. Go all the way up and all the way down in perfect style. Another tip that might help you in your quest to build classic calves is to concentrate on having all of the pressure or weight on your big toe. A lot of people do calf raises with their toes pointing out, and then they do them with their toes pointing ahead, and then — finally — with their toes pointing inwards. You don't need to do all of that. In fact, doing that is a waste of time! All you have to do is point your toes straight ahead and put 90 percent of all the weight on the big toe as you go up and down.

Isolating the Deltoids

Question: You mentioned earlier that one should try to avoid overdeveloping their trapezius muscles. Are there ways to still train your shoulders and not have it affect their traps?

Steve Reeves: There certainly are. As mentioned, if you overdevelop your trapezius or "traps" muscle you will cultivate a "round-shouldered" look. One method to target your delts and effectively remove your traps is to lock your lats when performing the upright row; flex them — hard — and concentrate on sustaining this fully-flexed position — while performing your upright rows. This act will serve to lock your scapulae and prevents you from raising your shoulders — effectively disengaging the trapezius from assisting in the movement — and thereby throwing the bulk of the training stress upon the muscle group you wish to develop maximally — your deltoids.

Training Partners

Question: What do you look for in a good training partner?

Steve Reeves: You look for a person who has enthusiasm, who is always up and somebody who is always prompt. You would also want somebody who encourages you but who doesn't ask of you the impossible. If you're supposed to do between seven and 11 reps, and you've just "run out of gas" on your ninth rep and you know that you couldn't hit 10 reps if someone offered you a million bucks, and he says, "Come on! Four more!" That's ridiculous.

A training partner should be able to know when to encourage you and when to shut up. When I worked out, I liked to concentrate deeply — I mean deeply — on the muscle I was training. I would visualize it growing and seeing the muscles, tendons and fibers working. I didn't want somebody to come up and say, "Hey Steve, how do you do this?" I had my workout partner trained so that when he saw someone coming over to interrupt my workout he'd say, "Hey look, he'll be happy to talk to you after his workout — or before his workout. He'll be happy to help you in any way he can, but during his workout, don't bug him. He wants to concentrate and get the most he can out of his workout while he's here."

I mean, I was there to do a job — as was my training partner. So good training partners look out for each other. And if you're workout partner is more or less the same strength as you, that's nice too.

Motivating Factors

Question: Did you ever do anything to "amp" your motivation for an upcoming contest?

Steve Reeves: Oh yes, particularly when I was training with Bob Wiedlick, who was a terrific training partner. I remember when I was training for the Mr. America contest, Bob, my training partner, would count my reps for me. I would always try to get at least 10 reps and he'd count: "One...two...three...four...five," and on the sixth rep he would begin to name some of the competitors that I'd be up against in the Mr. America contest. I knew who they were, but they had never seen me because I didn't want my pictures in the magazines before entering the contest. So what Bob did was start saying their names. These were the guys I knew I had to beat to win the contest, so instead of reps number "six, seven, eight, nine and ten" the reps became "Eiferman, Farbotnik, Pederson, Joe Lauriano and Kimon Voyages." In fact, they were in the top six when I won. Using that substitution of people for numbers would really motivate me to train hard in my workouts.

Training Equipment Advances

Question: What is your opinion of the advances made in exercise machines in training; for example, Universal, Cybex and Nautilus?

Steve Reeves: Well, I don't know if they're "advances" or not, but they certainly provide an alternative to free weights. I guess the greatest advance of those machines is that they're safer for the average person to use. Whereas with free weights, a person might drop them on himself or sustain an injury, these machines have a safety factor built into them. That's their greatest advantage. I would like to add that versatility is another plus. The machines — such as the Universal Gym system that I presently have at home — provide resistance where there wouldn't be any otherwise in the form of variable resistance. For instance, when you lift a barbell it's either hard or medium or easy at various points in the range of motion; but with a machine you get difficult resistance spread evenly all the way up and all the way down. The greatest advantage of the machines had been the introduction of variable resistance to training.

Pulley Power!

Question: I understand you are a big advocate of training with wall pulleys. Why is that?

Steve Reeves: I really like pulleys. I think with pulleys you get greater resistance spread over a greater range of motion than with barbells. I like pulleys a lot. In fact, a person can get a complete workout on pulleys and not have to do anything else! They're just that efficient — if you have them set up right. And by set up right I mean that it's important to use cross-pulleys. Have a room that's about 12-feet wide, a pulley on one wall and a pulley on the opposite wall, so that you can do all sorts of "crossing" exercises for your shoulders, chest and back.

Building a Classic Physique — on an Exercise Machine

Question: As many of us don't belong to a commercial gym, but have a home gym machine — as opposed to free weights — is there a way that we can build a classic physique utilizing the training principles you've espoused, but on an exercise machine?

Steve Reeves: I would say that if you have an exercise machine like Global or Universal, a multi-station machine, then you should do the same exercises that I recommend, except use your machine instead of the barbells or other pulleys. The beauty of these machines is that everything is there; stations to do your bench presses using a wide or narrow grip; chins, overhead presses, leg work, overhead pulley, low pulley and so on. Basically, you can do everything you need to do on one of these machines. And, although a basic Universal machine only has a leg press station to train your legs — as opposed to the various types of squats I recommend — you can still get much benefit from using this station properly. It's a great station and it's on the right angle. And, sitting there with those hand grips on the side, you can really concentrate on what you're doing — you don't have to worry about your balance as you would, say, in performing squats.

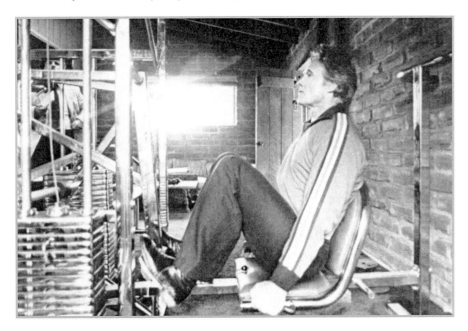

Steve Reeves' Current Training Program

Question: Since you now train at home on your ranch on a Universal machine, and are still having great workouts, and are still in great shape, could you tell us what your present training program consists of?

Steve Reeves: I mainly use wall pulleys along with certain select exercise stations

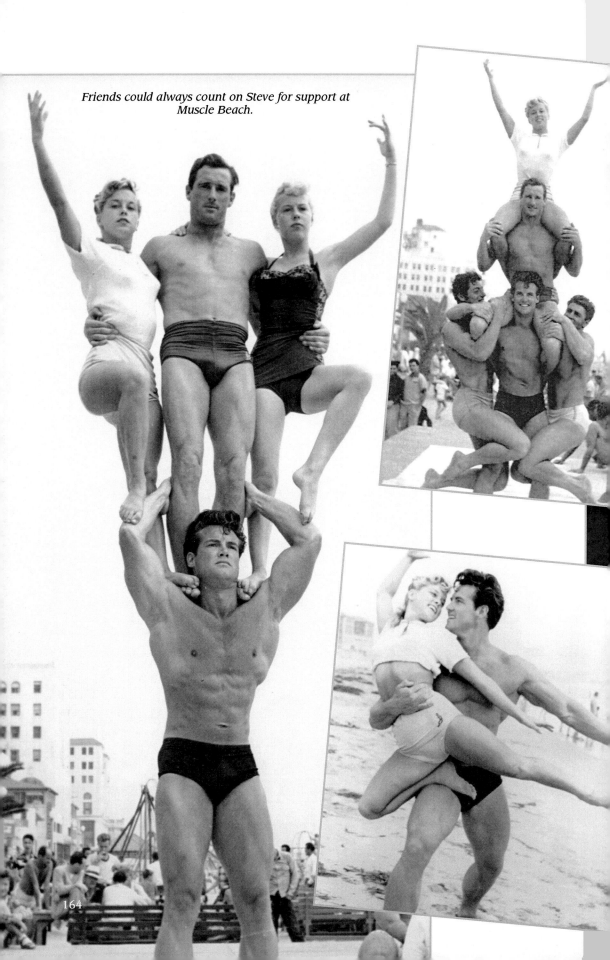

Friends could always count on Steve for support at Muscle Beach.

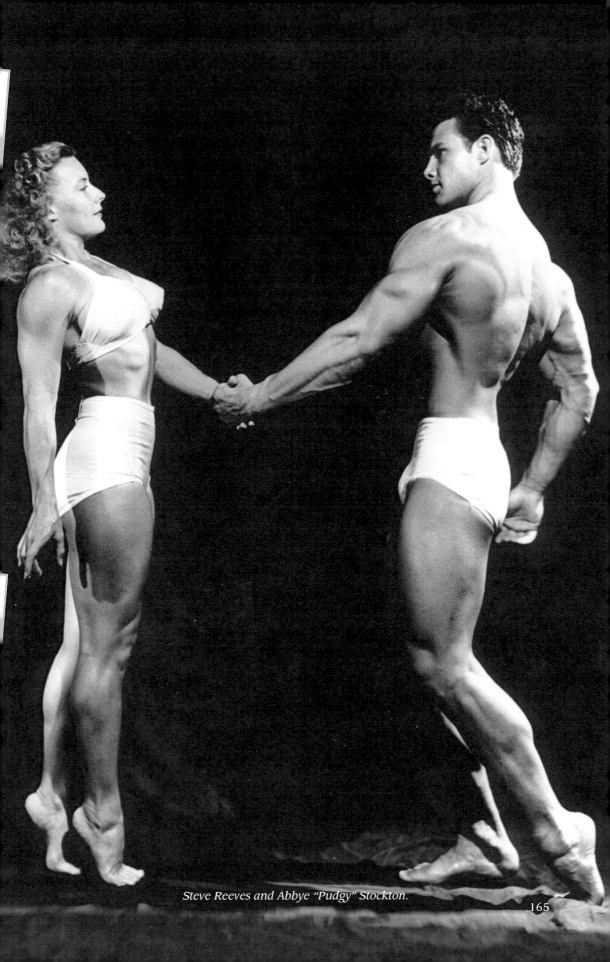
Steve Reeves and Abbye "Pudgy" Stockton.

from my Universal machine. I have my wall pulleys mounted on walls 12 feet apart, so I can do a lot of crossover pulley work.

In any event, I start out by doing upright rowing using one set of wall pulleys, holding the handles that are attached to the low pulleys. My right hand will be pulling on a cable that is attached to the left pulley and my left hand will be pulling on a cable that is attached to the pulley on the right. I make it a point to have the cables cross over in front of me. In this fashion, instead of simply pulling straight up, I'm able to pull up and out on an angle, which gets the deltoids even more effectively, I've found.

I've calmed down a bit in my training since I've turned 70 — but just a bit, mind you! I'm now performing only two sets of each exercise instead of three. In any event, after my upright rows, I'll move on to overhead presses for another two sets, and then finish off with two sets of lateral raises while lying back on a flat bench. I'll lie down on my bench on my back and take a pulley from each wall in the opposite hand, so that they're crossed over my chest — and then draw them across my chest until my hands are as far apart from one another as they can be. This is really good movement for the rear deltoid head and there's absolutely no way for me to cheat on the movement. I'm effectively pinned against the bench and can only move the handles by going all the way down and all the way up in a smooth, controlled movement.

I actually prefer pulleys to free-weights in this respect; you get a effective level of resistance over a greater range of motion. With a free weight, the first one-quarter of the movement is easy; the next half is hard and the last quarter is easy. With pulleys, if you get them on the right angle, they provide a constant level of resistance all the way up. This gives you greater benefit while putting in less time in the gym.

After completing the deltoid training, I move into chest work, beginning with the bench press station on the Universal. I perform two sets using a flat bench; one set with a wide grip, and the second set with a medium grip. Then I'll perform one inclined set of bench presses on a special incline bench I have. Then I end up doing crossover pulley work in the reverse fashion of how I performed my deltoid laterals. I hold a handle in each hand that is connected to a base pulley on the wall closest to the handle. (I don't cross the pulleys over this time. Unlike dumbbells, where it's hard from beginning to midpoint and then easy from the midpoint to the finish, with cables you get resistance in that last quarter of the movement that you don't get with dumbbells, thereby providing effective resistance over another foot and a half of motion.

After completing chest training, I do some lat work, using the pulldown-behind-neck movement on the high pulley and low-pulley-seated rowing. Next I move on to lower back and do hyperextensions on a little machine I made. This hits my lower back directly. To increase the resistance on this movement, I sometimes hang a 20-pound belt filled with lead around my neck and perform one set of 30 repetitions. I am doing less weight and more reps, now that I am older. I'm up to 15 reps normally, for most of my exercises. For muscles such as legs, I'll do 25 reps, and for the back, 30 reps.

I think when you get to a certain point in life, it's important to keep up the really good motion so you lower your weight and increase your reps. I find that I'm hitting some muscle fibers with this type of training that I never hit before.

Basically, scientific training is the amount of resistance, the duration in between and intervals. In other words, the amount of weight, the time it takes you to do it, and the intervals in between. And intervals of rest also. So the amount of weight you use, let's say you use 50 pounds twenty times, or 70 pounds ten times — it's the same effect. I find when you get older, your tendons, ligaments and joints might not be as limber or as strong as they were at one time, so why stress them? If you're doing 15 reps, it's easier to get that last rep in than it is if you're doing seven or eight reps with a heavier weight.

After hyperextensions, I'll move on to biceps using the incline bench curl with floor pulleys. I have a special bar that has a three-point contact. The two floor pulleys then attach to a cable I had built that is attached to the handle and it allows me to really focus on contracting my biceps without worrying about balancing the handle, as you do when you're curling up against, say, one cable. It's really smooth. That's all I do for biceps — I'll do two sets of those.

For triceps, I kneel in front of the wall pulley machine and grab hold of a bar with a revolving sleeve on it and just do some pulley pushdowns. I make sure that I'm in really close to the machine so that all three heads of the triceps are activated upon complete contraction. The reason I kneel is that it's better for the pulley work. The weights go up and down smoother than when you're standing up, and you can't cheat as much. It's a better way to isolate the muscle, relax and do it well. Then I move on to abdominals, where I'll perform 50 reps of knee-ups at the special knee-up station on the Universal machine with five pounds around each ankle. However, I've redesigned the knee-up backboard because it was perfectly vertical — which places far too much stress on your lower back — and I've reclined it a little. Now it works perfectly, allowing me to really target my abdominals.

I don't do anything for calves. But for legs, generally I go to the leg press station on the Universal machine and select a weight that I can press out 25 times with the adjustable chair moved out fairly far from the machine. For my second set, I move the seat in considerably and raise the weight and do another set. I pyramid my weights here — going light, heavy and light again. I warm up with the first set, then do a heavy set, and finally a light set at the end, just after the heavy set with the seat further forward. This way the tendons, ligaments and joints are all warmed up, so I can go deeper without the possibility of injury.

I know a lot of guys over the age of 50 are walking around with bad knees, bad hips and bad backs because they tried to use too much weight, too soon when they were working out — or they didn't take the time to warm up correctly — or both. So it's very important to warm up.

I finish my workout with thrusts using the wall pulleys. Thrusts are a great exercise for your glutes and abs. I attach a cable to the two lower pulleys of one wall pulley machine. I attach a strong belt — about two inches wide — to the other end of the cable. I adjust the belt so that it rests over my hip bones. I take a firm stance, placing my feet 12 to 18 inches apart and about 18-inches back from the pulley. Holding on to the pulley for support, I thrust my hips as far forward as possible and then let my hips return to a position as far back as I can go. I repeat my forward thrust for as many reps as I can in good form. Starting out, I used a weight that was approximately half of my bodyweight. If you wish to try this movement, you may want to simply use a weight with which you can complete 25 reps in good style.

Additional Training Considerations for the Older Bodybuilder

Question: Is there any particular advice that you have for older bodybuilders? Any advice you would give them when they are just starting out?

Steve Reeves: I would say to get a medical check up first. Then if you're just starting

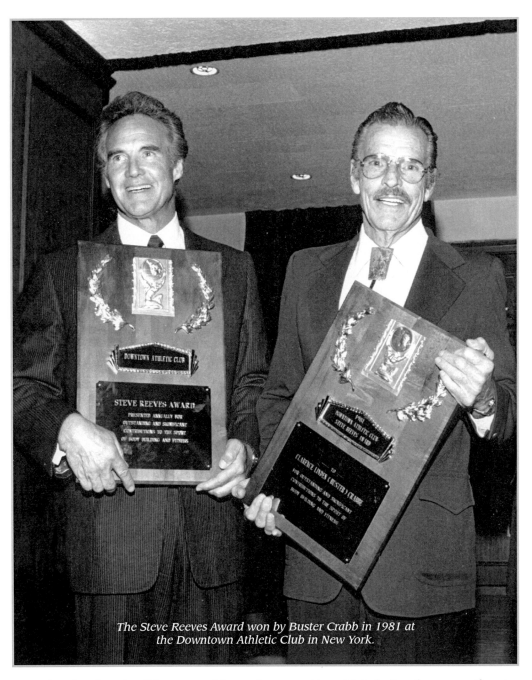

The Steve Reeves Award won by Buster Crabb in 1981 at the Downtown Athletic Club in New York.

to work out and you're, 50 years or older and you want to get into better shape—or, if you're a person who has been working out for years and wants to stay in shape, all you need is to do three sets per muscle group. You don't need nine sets. I would say that an ideal routine for anybody — whether young or old — is to workout three days per week but have the maximum amount of rest in between your workouts.

For example, you would train Monday morning, Wednesday night and Saturday morning. With this schedule, you get yourself another 12 hours or so of rest. Of, if you can't do that, you can workout Monday night, Thursday morning and Saturday night. That way you have a prolonged rest in between workouts to recuperate and to balance the training.

If I were to workout hard again or really try to shape up fast, gain size and so on, this is the schedule I would follow. It has just the right amount of time to recuperate. However, Monday, Wednesday and Friday are also fine, as you have Saturday and Sunday to rest. But sometimes if you rest too long, it becomes hard to get started again. And it may be that those 48-hours you have between workouts might not be enough. Maybe 60-hours would have been better. I think that's the ideal routine for the older trainee.

Greatest Influences

Question: Who were your greatest influences in bodybuilding?

Steve Reeves: Well, that's hard to say. When I first started training I used to look at pictures of different bodybuilders, but there was never any one particular bodybuilder that made me think, "Gee, I want to be like him." For instance, I would look at John Grimek and say, "You know I'd like to have legs like that — now there's a good pair of legs. Grimek has calves and thighs that balance. I'd like to have a pair of legs like Grimek's." Then I'd look at Al Stephan and I'd say: "Now there's a great pair of lats. What a back!"

I'd like to have legs like Grimek, lats like Stephan, arms like Sam Loprinzi and definition like Clarence Ross, with a great taper from chest to waist like Jack LaLanne — who had a 20-inch differential in this regard — and that's the way I'd do it. I would just be making a composite of these different bodybuilders. But looking back, I would have to say that Ed Yarick, my mentor and trainer, was my greatest influence.

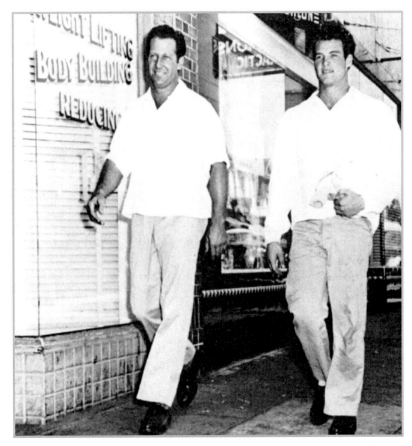

Steve with Ed Yarick in front of Ed's gym at 13550 Foothill Boulevard, Oakland, 1947.

The Importance of Genetics

Question: How important are genetics in building a classic physique?

Steve Reeves: I think genetics are very important and they certainly have a lot to do with the ultimate success you will achieve in bodybuilding. I mean, if you don't have the materials, how can you build the house? You might have to settle for a well-structured cabin.

DNA as a Limiting Factor?

Question: Do you feel that an individual can only improve so much — and then that's it? I mean, does DNA somehow limit your ultimate potential?

Steve Reeves: Well there is a limit, yes. But you can off-balance that limit by having deep concentration and making sure that you have all the necessary amino acids in your diet along with the proper vitamins and minerals. In other words, a person who has great potential — genetically — but who doesn't eat correctly and doesn't train properly, can be outclassed by a person who has less genetic potential but who does everything correctly.

It's true in any sport — not just bodybuilding. Look at an athlete like Pete Rose; I mean he was out there giving 110 percent all the time. He was a good athlete but he wasn't really "gifted." He excelled because he wanted to. He had concentration! Whereas another ball player who'd always been good, might have gotten only by giving 90 percent — but his 90 percent wasn't as good as Rose's 110 percent, if you know what I mean.

Acquiring a Deep Tan

Question: I suppose that living in California as you do would allow you to acquire a wonderful tan — and thereby really showcase your physique. However, was there anything special that you did before a contest to deepen your tan?

Steve Reeves: Well, and some people may laugh at this, I would eat a lot of iron — in the form of raisins — and drink a lot of carrot juice. The reason I did this was that having iron in your system makes your skin a little reddish — a blush color — while carrot juice makes you a little orangish. So with the red and orange together — combined with a little sun — I'd always end up with a real brilliant tan.

Shaving Down

Question: Did you have to shave your body hair in order to compete in bodybuilding contests, like the rest of the pros do today?

Steve Reeves: Yes, all bodybuilders shave down in order to prevent the hair from obstructing the judges' view of their muscles. I used to shave down with an electric razor perhaps one week before the event — sometimes only two days before so that I'd be close shaved. They were electric razors such as you see advertised in some catalogues now, but in my day we could only get them from barber shops.

The Subject of Steroids

Question: What are your thoughts on the steroid issue in bodybuilding?

Steve Reeves: I think the introduction of steroids was the worst thing to ever happen to bodybuilding. To me, the bodybuilders of today look like clones. They all look like they're out of the same mold. Sure, some of them have blond hair, others dark hair, some have fair skin, others dark skin and some are shorter and some are taller, but all of them look like they were stamped out of the same mold. And that's the sort of bloated-tissue look caused by steroids. In my day, from 100 yards away, you could tell if a person was Steve Reeves or John Grimek, Clancy Ross or Reg Park. People were individuals at that time. Now they workout with the same routine, with the same steroids, and as a result, they've come to look too much like one another.

They waste their lives training all the time. There's more to life than training. And when they're off the drugs, they don't look that great. Contrast that with John Grimek — I saw John about six months ago — at age 85 — and he's still looking good! In my day, bodybuilding was a health-oriented activity — instead of the drug-oriented sport it has since become. Steroids surfaced in bodybuilding, I think, because people wanted to take the "easy way" to get to the top. Then, when one guy took the easy way and got results, somebody else did it and it just snowballed from there. Even the judges encouraged it by giving out trophies to people with the "biggest" legs — not the "best developed legs" — the "biggest arms, not the "best developed" arms, and so on. I just think it got out of hand. If everybody got off steroids, I think the quality of physiques would improve because all of the athletes would be competing at a body weight that would be, more or less, ideal for their individual frames.

More on Steroids

Question: The other day at the local library I was looking at a book entitled, "Arnold: An Unauthorized Biography" by an author named Wendy Leigh. On page 27 it stated that Kurt Marnul told Arnold [Schwarzenegger] about steroids. Marnul said that he had learned about steroids and their dosage from Steve Reeves, whom he claims to have met in France during a 1952 vacation. Is this true?

Steve Reeves: That statement has also been brought to my attention by a friend who surfs the Internet. No it is not true. I never heard of steroids until the mid 1960s and I was never in France during the 1950s! My first trip to France was in 1948 when I entered and won the "Mr. World" contest in Cannes. My second trip to France was not until 1960 when I attended the premiere of my movie, *The Last Days Of Pompeii*.

I have never heard of Kurt Marnul and I don't know what motive he had in making that statement to Arnold. I can only speculate that he might have mixed me up with another bodybuilder of that period, or that he was trying to impress Arnold by telling him that he knew me.

A Word on Definitions

Question: I notice that you don't utilize common bodybuilding terms like "stressing the muscles" or "overloading the muscles." Why is that?

Steve Reeves: You're quite correct, and the reason is because I don't think they are accurate terms to describe the actual training process. To me, the term "stress" connotes something negative, or something to be avoided. In which case, I prefer to use "increased demands" — which is what you are asking your muscles to accomplish in a given workout. The same holds true with terms like "overload." To my way of thinking if you truly were to "overload" something, you would break it — which makes it a thing to avoid. With regard to increasing the demands placed on your muscles, however, I think the term "maxi-load" would be more adequate, as it implies the maximum amount of load or demand that a muscle is capable of contracting against in good form. These definitions help to put me in

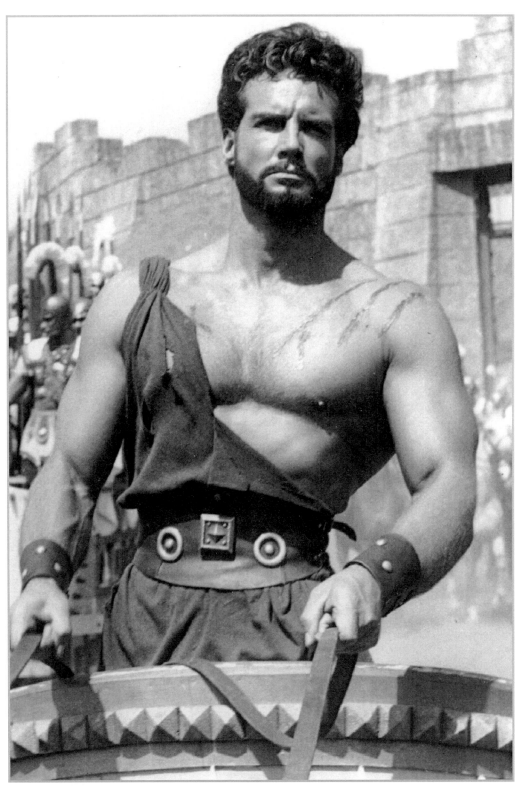

Some of Steve's memorable movie roles: above and near right, "Hercules" released by Warner Brothers in 1959; top opposite page, "Goliath and the Barbarians" in 1960; and bottom opposite page, "The Slave, Son of Spartacus" in 1963.

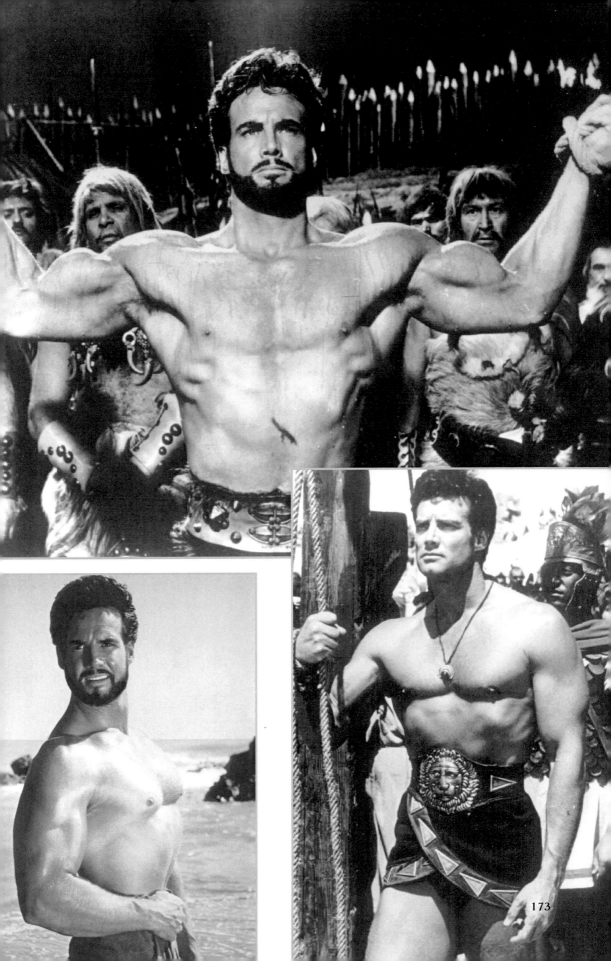

the proper mind-set when I train, and also reinforce the fact that bodybuilding — properly performed — is not about stress and negativity, but positive, good old-fashioned hard work.

PHILOSOPHY OF LIFE

Question: What philosophy of life or integrated view of human existence do you subscribe to?

Steve Reeves: Well, my philosophy of life is to be able to function well regardless of your means. In other words, to be able to adjust. I can live in a palace and be very comfortable or I can live in a tent somewhere in the outdoors, enjoying nature in the fresh air.

You shouldn't have too many material expectations in life. You should always try to lead a balanced life. Don't be a fanatic in any way, and always have a positive attitude.

A TYPICAL DAY

Question: What does a typical day consist of these days for Steve Reeves?

Steve Reeves: Well, I get up around 6 a.m. and I have the same thing to eat every morning. I'll have a tall glass of orange juice — freshly squeezed from oranges that I've picked off my own trees on the ranch, and stir in a tablespoon of honey and I take some bee pollen tablets. That gets my energy up. Then I'll take a lengthy bicycle ride or a Power Walk, then work out in my home gym for 30 to 40 minutes; shower, then lie down for a half an hour.

Rising, I have my Power Drink, then go out to ride and train my horses for about an hour. Then, I do a little work in the garden or on the fruit trees around the ranch. I'll have lunch at 12:30 p.m., and at 1 p.m. I'll take a nap. I'm up at 2:30 p.m. and go for a ride on another horse for about an hour. When I return, I go to my desk to do what business needs to be done, watch the news, do some reading — and that's the day.

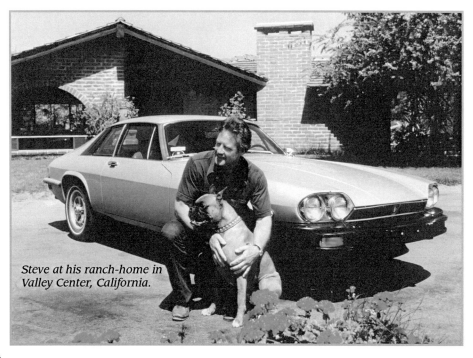

Steve at his ranch-home in Valley Center, California.

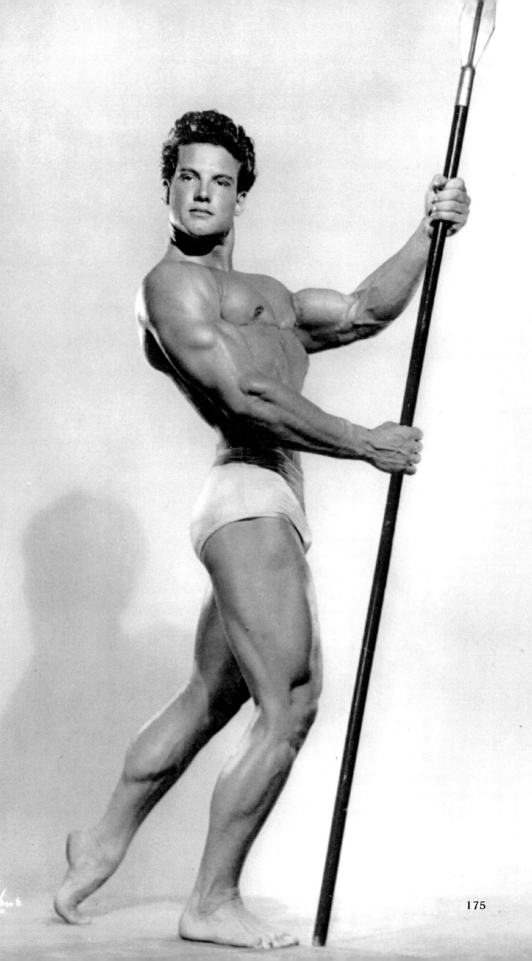

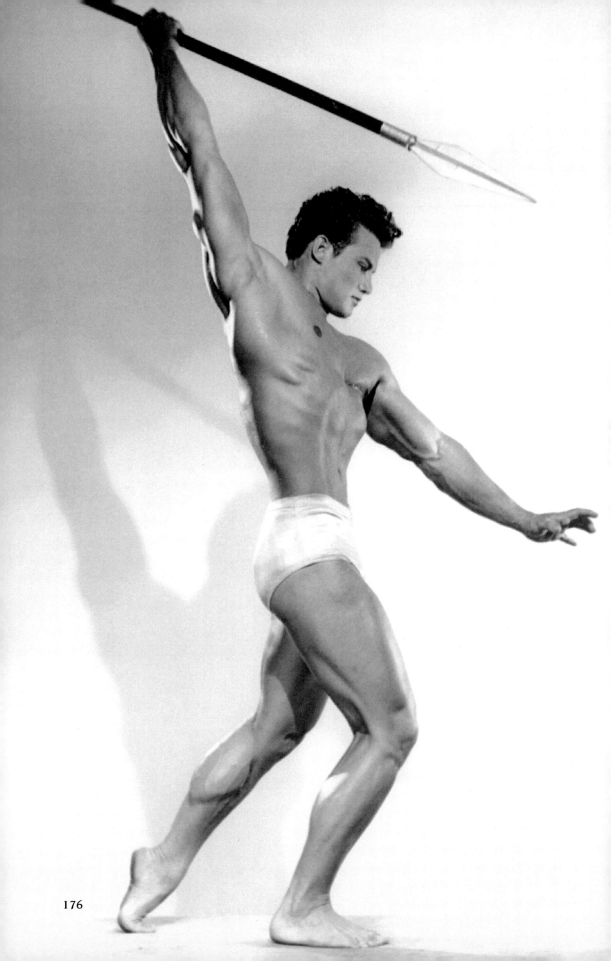

Appendix 1

My Championship Workout

This is the course I used when I trained for the Mr. America and Mr. Universe Contests.

Upright Rowing — 3 sets — 8-12 reps.
  Barbell - narrow grip -

Press Behind Neck — 3 sets — 8-12 reps.
  Barbell - wide grip -

Lateral Raises — 3 sets — 8-12 reps.
  Dumbbells - bent over -

Bench Press — 3 sets — 8-12 reps.
  Barbell - wide grip -

Incline Bench Press — 3 sets — 8-12 reps.
  Dumbbells - thumbs in -

Flying Motion — 3 sets — 8-12 reps.
  Dumbbells - bent armed -

Pulldowns Behind Neck — 3 sets — 8-12 reps
  Overhead Pulley - wide grip -

Rowing Seated   3 sets.   8-12 reps.
    Lat Pulley – narrow grip –

One Arm Rowing   3 sets.   8-12 reps.
    Dumbell – pull back toward hips –

Incline Bench Curl   6 sets   5-7 reps.
    Dumbells – working down the rack –

Bench Curl   3 sets   8-12 reps.
    Overhead Pulley – bar –

Concentration Curls   1 set.   8-12 reps
    Dumbell – elbow resting on inside of knee –

Tricep Pushdowns   3 sets   8-12 reps.
    High Pulley – narrow –

Tricep Extensions   3 sets   8-12 reps.
    One Dumbell – behind neck –

Tricep Crossovers   3 sets   8-12 reps.
    Dumbell – one arm, lying on bench –

Parallel Squats   3 sets   8-12 reps
    Barbell – heels on 2" block –

Hack Lifts   2 sets   8-12 Reps
Barbell   - heels on block -

Front Squate   2 sets   8-12
Barbell   - held in clean position -

Leg Curls   2 sets   8-12
    - resistance by workout partner

Calf Raises   3 sets   20-25
Leg press machine

Forward bends   3 sets   12-15
Barbell   - seated on bench -

Knee Raises   2 sets   20-25
Vertical Bench   - ankle weights -

Work neck   1 set   15-20
all four sides - Resistance by workout
Partner.

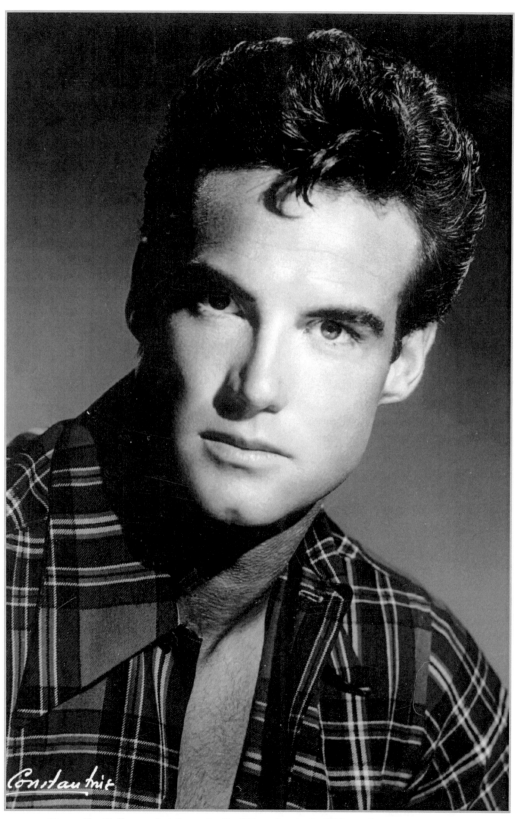

Dramatic, Hollywood-style portrait of Steve to start off his acting career — 1952.

APPENDIX 2

My Favorite Bodybuilding Exercises

DELTOIDS
1. Upright Rowing (barbell)
2. Press-Behind-Neck (wide-grip, barbell)
3. Military Press (barbell)
4. Alternate Press (dumbbells)
5. Alternate Front Raises (dumbbells)
6. Bent-Over Lateral Raises (dumbbells)
7. Lateral Raises (dumbbells)
8. Upright Rowing (wall pulley)
9. Incline Front Raises (wall pulley)
10. Laterals on Bench (wall pulley)

CHEST
1. Bench Press (barbell)
2. Bench Press (wide-grip, barbell)
3. Bench Press (dumbbells)
4. Incline Press (barbell)
5. Incline Press (dumbbells)
6. Flying Motion (dumbbells)
7. Laterals (dumbbells)
8. Laterals (wall pulley)
9. Pec Crossover (wall pulley)
10. Parallel Bar Dip (with weight belt)

LATISSIMUS
1. Straight-Arm Pullover (barbell)
2. Pulldown-Behind-Neck (high pulley)
3. Bent-Over Rowing (barbell)
4. Bent-Arm Pullover (barbell)
5. One-Arm Row (dumbbell)
6. Incline Pullover (wall pulley, bar)
7. T-Bar Rowing (barbell)
8. Low-Pulley Rowing (handles, low pulley)
9. Pull-Up Behind Neck (wide-grip, high bar)
10. Lat Stretch (upright support)

BICEPS
1. Curl Standing (barbell)
2. Incline Bench Curl (dumbbells)
3. Preacher Curl (barbell)
4. Alternate Curl (dumbbell)
5. Reverse Curl (barbell)
6. Crucifix Curl (wall pulley)
7. Wall-Pulley Curl (wall pulley)
8. High-Pulley Bench-Curl (high pulley)
9. Concentration Curl (dumbbell)
10. Incline Bench-Curl (wall pulley)

TRICEPS
1. Press Down (bar, high pulley)
2. Incline Triceps Extension (palms-in, dumbbells)
3. Triceps Extension Bench Press (thumbs-in, barbell)
4. Triceps Extension Bench Press (palms-in, dumbbells)
5. One-Arm Cross Over (dumbbell)
6. Triceps Extension Behind Neck (one arm, dumbbell)
7. Triceps Extension Bench Press (thumbs-out, barbell)
8. Triceps Extension Wall Pulley (facing away, wall pulley w/handles)
9. Bent-Over Triceps Extension (dumbbells or wall pulley w/handles)
10. Press Down (kneeling, wall pulley w/bar handle)

LEGS
1. Squat (parallel, barbell)
2. Front Squat (barbell)
3. Hack Lift (barbell)
4. Lunge (dumbbells)
5. Leg Curl (machine)
6. Leg Extension (machine)

CALVES
1. Calf Raise Standing (machine or barbell)
2. Calf Raise Seated (barbell)
3. Donkey-Calf Raise (workout partner)
4. One-Leg Calf Raise (dumbbell)

Note: Always do your calf raises on a board three to four inches high.

LOWER BACK
1. Deadlift (barbell)
2. Forward Bend (seated on bench, barbell)
3. Forward Bend (twisting, barbell)
4. Back Raise (high bench, dumbbell)

ABDOMINALS
1. Bent Knee Curl-Up (bodyweight)
2. Leg Raise (no resistance)
3. Crunch (no resistance)
4. Knee-Up (horizontal station, with weight belt)
5. Thrust (wall pulley)

My Favorite Bodybuilding Exercises -- *in detail*

Warm-Up

Dumbbell Swing Through

The motion consists of grasping a light dumbbell (start out with 10 pounds) and, with your feet spread a little wider than shoulder-width apart, bend at the knees and place the dumbbell between your legs and as far behind you as possible.

From this position, straighten to a standing position as you swing the dumbbell upward and over your head as far as you can reach. Immediately return to the starting position and repeat.

The dumbbell swing is a great total-body warm-up exercise that will really prepare your muscles for the workout to come.

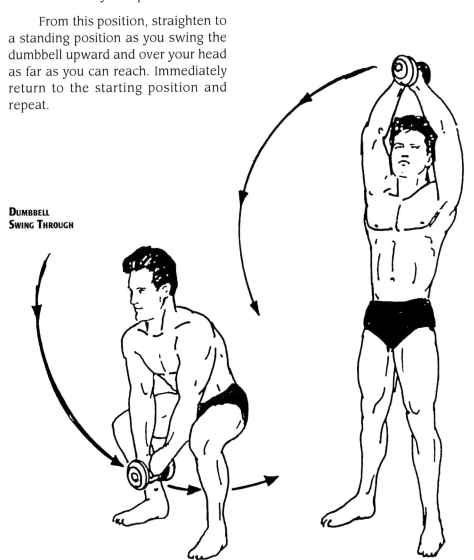

DUMBBELL SWING THROUGH

Illustrations by Jim Dallmeier

Deltoids

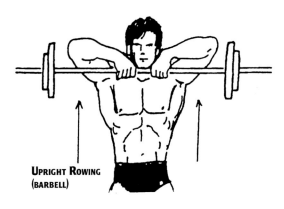

Upright Rowing (Barbell)

Stand with your feet about 12-inches apart. Grasp the barbell with your hands six inches apart with your "thumbs-in." Pull the weight up smoothly until it nearly touches your chin, keeping your elbows out. Pause. Then lower the weight slowly to the starting position. Repeat.

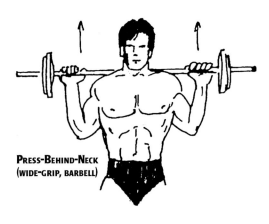

Press-Behind-Neck (Wide-Grip, Barbell)

Stand with your feet about 12-inches apart. Grasp the barbell with your "thumbs-in." Clean the weight to your shoulders. Press overhead. Then lower to the back of your head letting it rest on your trapezius. Now take a wide grip on the bar. Press overhead in a smooth movement. Pause before lowering the weight slowly to the starting position. Repeat.

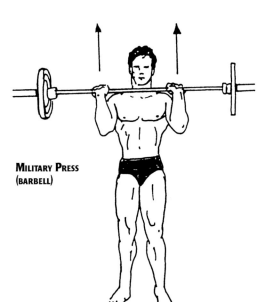

Military Press (Barbell)

Stand with your feet about 12-inches apart. Grasp the barbell with your hands at shoulder-width using the "thumbs-in" position. Clean the weight and press it smoothly overhead. Then slowly lower it to the starting position. Repeat.

Incline Alternate Front Raises (Dumbbells)

Lie on an incline bench with a dumbbell in each hand. Utilizing the "thumbs-in" position, raise one dumbbell overhead. As you slowly lower this dumbbell, raise the dumbbell in the other hand. Repeat alternating raises until you finish the set.

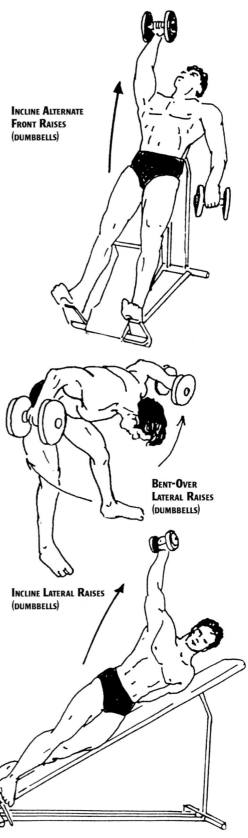

Bent-Over Lateral Raises (Dumbbells)

Stand with your feet about 18-inches apart. Grab a pair of dumbbells and bend forward at the waist. Using the "palms-in" position with your arms slightly bent, raise the weights smoothly out to your sides and up until they are parallel to the floor. Hold for a moment. Then lower slowly to the starting position. Repeat.

Incline Lateral Raises (Dumbbells)

Lie on your side on an incline bench with a dumbbell in one hand in the "palm-down" position. Raise the dumbbell smoothly overhead. Pause. Lower it slowly to the starting position. Repeat.

Chest

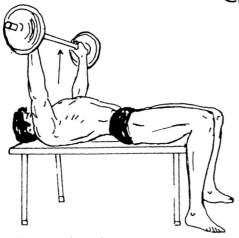

BENCH PRESS (BARBELL)

Bench Press (Wide-grip, Barbell)

Lie with your back on the bench and your feet on the floor. Using a grip of approximately 18-inches wider than your shoulders, press the barbell smoothly to arm's length over your chest. With a momentary pause, slowly lower the barbell to your chest. Repeat.

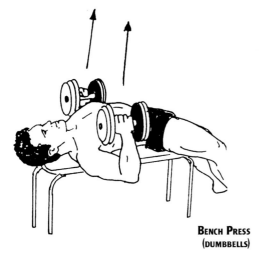

BENCH PRESS (DUMBBELLS)

Bench Press (Dumbbells)

Lie on the bench with a dumbbell in each hand. Using the "palms-in" position, press dumbbells overhead and lower to the sides of your chest. Repeat.

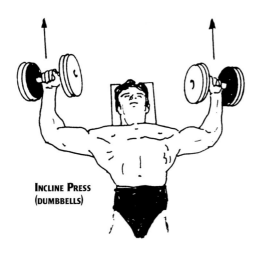

INCLINE PRESS (DUMBBELLS)

Incline Press (Dumbbells)

Lie on an incline bench with two dumbbells. Press the dumbbells to arm's length. With your palms facing forward, lower the dumbbells down and out until they are parallel to the floor. Your arms will be at right angles. Repeat.

Flying Motion

Lie on the bench with two dumbbells. Press dumbbells overhead. With a "thumbs-in" position and arms slightly bent, lower the dumbbells until they are lower than the bench. While still maintaining a slight bend in your arms, raise to starting position above your head. Repeat.

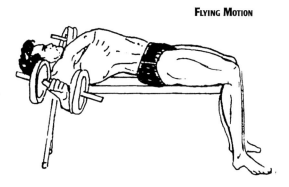

Laterals (Dumbbells)

Lie back on the bench with two dumbbells. Press dumbbells overhead. Using a "palms-in" position with arms straight, lower the dumbbells below the level of the bench. Keeping your arms straight, raise dumbbells above your head. Repeat.

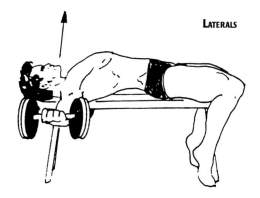

Parallel Bar Dip

Position yourself on the parallel bars. While concentrating on your lower pectorals, press yourself up. Keep you elbows close to your sides. Bend your arms, lowering your body as far as you can comfortably. Then press yourself up again until elbows are locked. Pause. Repeat.

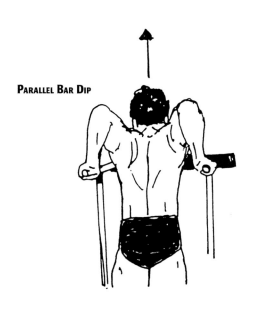

Latissimus

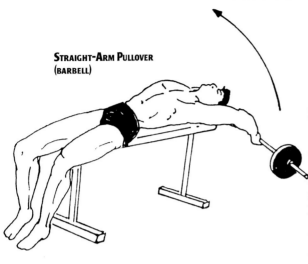

Straight-Arm Pullover (Barbell)

Straight-Arm Pullover (Barbell)

While holding the barbell, lie back on the bench. With hands approximately shoulder-width apart and "thumbs-in," press the weight overhead. While keeping your arms straight, lower the barbell down and back until it is parallel to the bench. Pause. Raise it back to the starting position. Repeat.

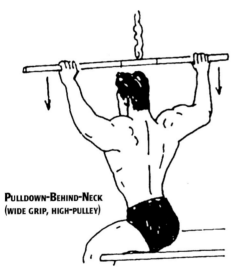

Pulldown-Behind-Neck (Wide Grip, High-Pulley)

Pulldown-Behind-Neck (Wide-Grip, High-Pulley)

Sit on the bench and take a wide grip on the overhead pulley bar. With "thumbs-in," pull the weight down to the back of your neck. Pause. Then resist the weight as you let it return to the starting position. Repeat.

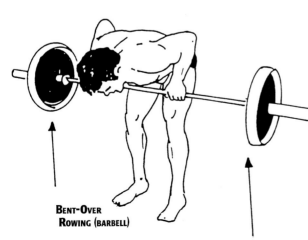

Bent-Over Rowing (Barbell)

Bent-Over Rowing (Barbell)

Stand with your feet about 18-inches apart. Using the "thumbs-in" position, grasp a barbell placing your hands approximately 24-inches apart. Bend over at the waist, keeping your legs slightly bent, and pull the weight up to your chest. Pause momentarily. Then lower the weight slowly to the starting position. Repeat.

Bent-Over Long Bar Rowing

Place your feet about 18-inches apart. Bend at the waist and grab the long bar with both hands just behind the plates. Pull the bar up to your chest. Pause. Then lower to the starting position. Repeat.

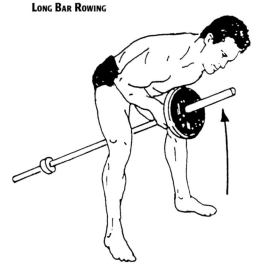

BENT-OVER LONG BAR ROWING

One-Arm Row (Dumbbell)

While supporting yourself on the bench, grab a dumbbell in the opposite hand. Keep your bench-side leg slightly bent and in front of the other leg (which should be kept straight). Pull the dumbbell up toward your hip, pause. Then lower to starting position. Switch sides and repeat.

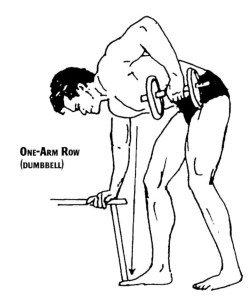

ONE-ARM ROW (DUMBBELL)

Low-Pulley Rowing

Sit on the floor and grip the handles of the low-pulleys with "palms-in." Bend slightly forward at the waist and pull the handle to your waist. While maintaining that position, resist the weight as you let it return to the starting position. Repeat.

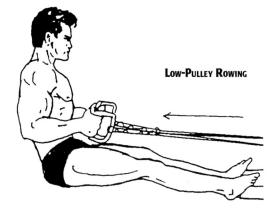

LOW-PULLEY ROWING

Biceps

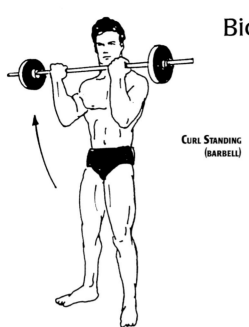
CURL STANDING (BARBELL)

Curl Standing (Barbell)

With your feet about shoulder-width apart, pick up the barbell. Using the "thumbs-out" position, curl the weight up to your chest. Make sure that you keep your elbows to your sides. Don't swing the barbell. Pause a moment, then lower the weight to the starting position. Repeat.

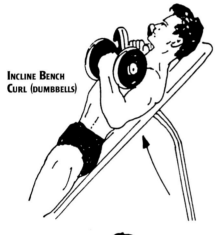
INCLINE BENCH CURL (DUMBBELLS)

Incline Bench Curl (Dumbbells)

Lie on an incline bench. Take hold of two dumbbells with a "thumbs-out" grip. While curling the dumbbells up to your chest, make sure you keep your elbows in and don't swing the weights. Pause at the top. Then slowly lower the weights to the starting position. Repeat.

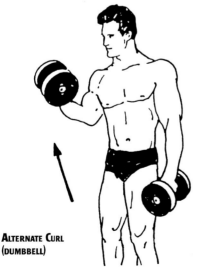
ALTERNATE CURL (DUMBBELL)

Alternate Curl (Dumbbells)

Take a pair of dumbbells off the rack, holding them in the "thumbs-out" position. Stand with your feet about 18-inches apart. Curl one dumbbell up to your shoulder. Pause. Then lower it slowly as you curl the other dumbbell up to your other shoulder. Repeat.

Reverse Curl (Barbell)

Grab a barbell in the "thumbs-in" position. Stand with your feet about 18-inches apart. Curl the weight up to your chest without swinging it. Pause. Then lower the weight slowly to the starting position. Repeat.

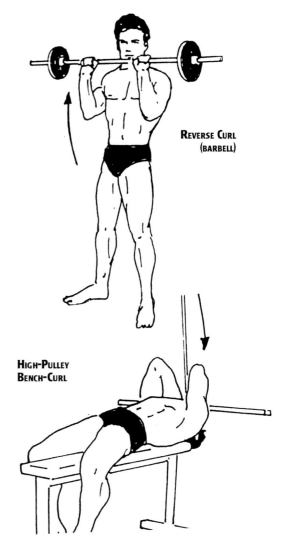

Reverse Curl (Barbell)

High-Pulley Bench-Curl

High-Pulley Bench-Curl

Place a bench under the high pulley. Lie on your back facing the pulley. Grab the bar with your hands approximately 12-inches apart in the "thumbs-out" position. Make sure the pulley is directly over your knees. While keeping your upper arms in place, curl the bar to your chin with a slow, smooth movement. Pause. Resist as you return to the starting position. Repeat.

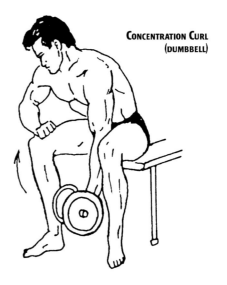

Concentration Curl (Dumbbell)

Concentration Curl (Dumbbell)

Grasp a dumbbell. Sit on a bench with the arm being worked resting against the inside of your knee in the "palms-up" position (rest the free hand on your other knee). Curl the weight smoothly up to your shoulder. Pause. Then slowly lower it down to the starting position. Repeat.

Triceps

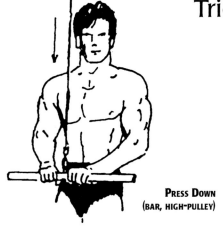

Press Down (Bar, High-Pulley)

Stand under an overhead pulley with your feet about 18-inches apart. Take a narrow grip on the bar. Make sure you keep your elbows in close and push the bar down. Pause. Resist the weight as you let it slowly return to the starting position. Repeat.

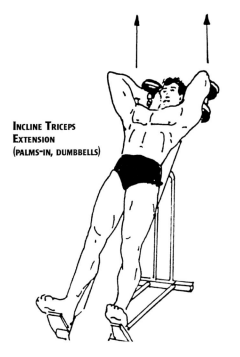

Incline Triceps Extension (Palms-In, Dumbbells)

Lie on an incline bench holding a pair of dumbbells with "palms-in." Press the weights overhead. Keeping your elbows in, lower the dumbbells down and back. Pause. Extend the dumbbells back to the overhead starting position. Repeat.

Triceps Extension Bench Press (Thumbs-In, Narrow-Grip, Barbell)

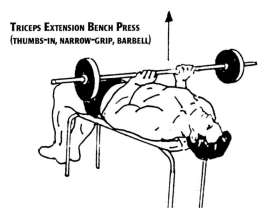

Lie on the bench holding a barbell with the "thumbs-in" and a narrow grip of about 12-inches. Press the weight over your chest. Pause. Then slowly lower the barbell to the starting position. Repeat.

One-Arm Cross Over (Dumbbell)

Holding one dumbbell, lie back on a bench. With a "thumbs-in" grip, extend the dumbbell above your chest. Use your other hand to support your upper arm and keep it still. Lower the weight across your body until it touches the opposite shoulder. Pause. Return to starting position. Repeat.

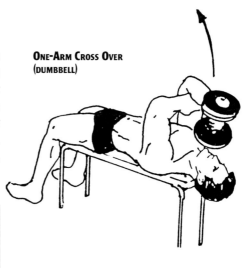

Triceps Extension Behind Neck (One Arm, Dumbbell)

Sit on bench. With one hand, hold a dumbbell in the "thumbs-in" position over your head. Lower the weight to behind your head. Pause. Without moving your elbow, extend the arm back to the starting position. Repeat.

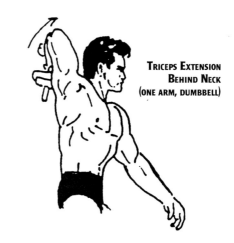

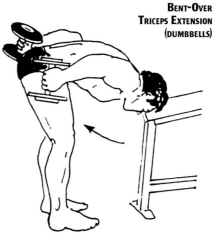

Bent-Over Triceps Extension (Dumbbells)

Grasp a pair of dumbbells. With your feet about shoulder-width apart, bend at the waist and rest your head on a high bench. Keep your upper arms parallel to your sides with your elbows held-in close. Extend the dumbbells back and up. Pause. Resist the weights as you return to the starting position. Repeat.

Legs

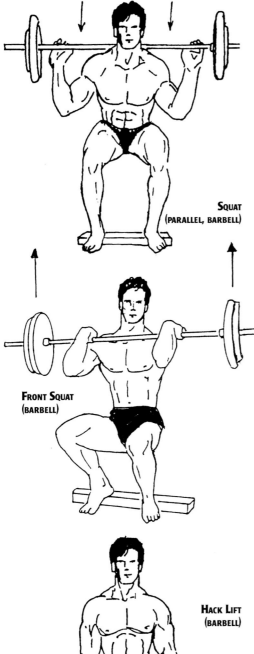

Squat (Parallel, Barbell)

Step under the squat rack. Hold a barbell across the back of your neck resting it on your trapezius. Balance the bar with your hands using a wide grip with "thumbs-in." Place your heels on a block two-to-three-inches high. Bend your knees and lower your body so that your legs are parallel to the floor. Pause. Return to the starting position. Repeat.

Front Squat (Barbell)

Grasp a barbell approximately shoulder-width with "thumbs-in." Clean and hold it in front of you resting the weight on the front of your deltoids and supporting it with your arms. Hold your elbows forward. Place your heels on a block two-to-three-inches thick with your feet 14 to 18-inches apart. Being careful to keep back straight, squat down past parallel. Pause. Return to the starting position. Repeat.

Lunge (Dumbbells)

Hold a dumbbell in each hand with "palms-in" and with your arms at your sides. Keeping your back straight, step forward with your right leg about two feet. While keeping your left leg as straight as possible, bend your knee until your thigh is parallel to the floor. Pause. Return to the starting position and repeat with your left leg.

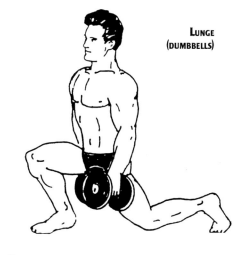

Leg Curl (Machine)

Lie face down on the bench of the leg extension machine. Place your heels under the rollers, making sure that your knees are slightly off the bench. Curl your legs up until the roller touches your buttocks. Pause. Lower your legs back to the starting position. Repeat.

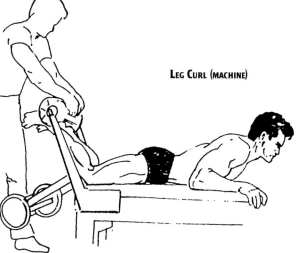

Leg Extension (Machine)

Sit at the end of the bench on the leg extension machine, with your knees bent. Place your feet under the rollers and extend your legs until they are straight. Pause. Lower your legs slowly to the starting position. Repeat.

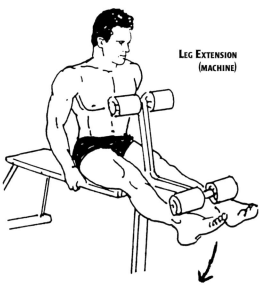

Calves

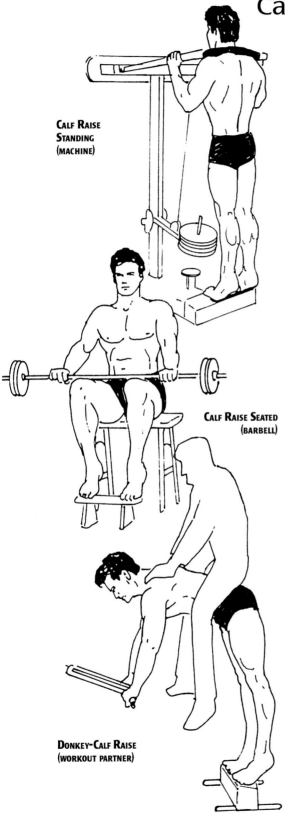

Calf Raise Standing (Machine)

Position your shoulders under the parallel extensions on the calf machine. Place your feet 12-inches apart on a three-to-four-inch thick block. Keep your back straight and your legs locked. Raise up as high as possible on the balls of your feet. Pause. Then lower your heels as far as possible to get a good stretch. Return to starting position. Repeat.

Calf Raise Seated (Barbell)

Sit on a bench with your feet positioned 12-inches apart on a three-to-four-inch thick block. Place a barbell on your thighs just above the knees. Raise up as high as possible on the balls of your feet. Pause. Then lower your heels as far as you can to get a good stretch. Return to the starting position. Repeat.

Donkey-Calf Raise (Workout Partner)

Place your feet 12-inches apart on a three-to-four-inch thick block. Keeping your legs straight, bend forward until your torso is parallel to the floor. Rest your hands on the bench. Have your buddy or workout partner sit on your lower back with the greater part of his/her weight supported by your hips. Keep your legs locked as you raise as high as possible on the balls of your feet. Pause, then lower your heels as far as possible to get a good stretch. Return to the starting position. Repeat.

Back

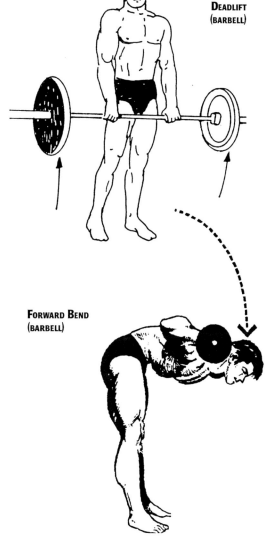

Deadlift (Barbell)

Place your feet about 18-inches apart with your knees bent. Reach down and grasp a barbell with your hands at shoulder-width and with "thumbs-in." Keeping your back straight, lift the weight by straightening your legs. Pause. Return to the starting position. Repeat.

Forward Bend (Barbell)

Place the barbell on the back of your neck resting on your trapezius. Hold the bar using the "thumbs-in" position and a wide grip. Keep your legs straight and bend forward at the waist until you are parallel to the floor. Pause. Return to the starting position. Repeat.

Back Raise

Using a high bench designed for this exercise, place your heels under the board and your upper body extending out over the pads supporting your upper thighs or groin. Bend downward at your waist until your torso is vertical to the floor. Pause. Then raise your upper body until it is past parallel with the floor. Repeat.

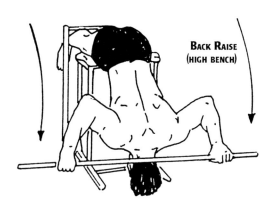

Abdominals

**BENT KNEE CURL-UP
(BODYWEIGHT)**

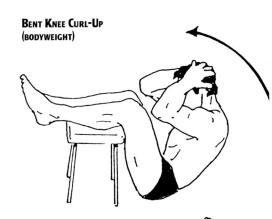

Bent Knee Curl-Up (Bodyweight)

Lie on the floor with your legs bent and calves resting on a low bench. Place your hands behind your neck and curl forward until your elbows touch your knees. Pause. Return to the starting position. Repeat.

**INCLINE ALTERNATE LEG RAISE
(NO RESISTANCE)**

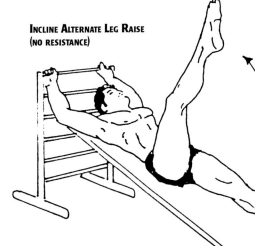

Incline Alternate Leg Raise (No Resistance)

Lie on the inclined abdominal board. Grip the rungs and raise your right leg up as high as comfortable. Pause. Then raise your left leg as you lower your right leg. Repeat.

KNEE-UP

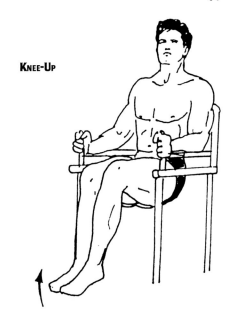

Knee-Up

Using the vertical bench, place your forearms on the armrests. Grip the handles while bracing your back against the backboard. Bend your legs as you raise your knees up to parallel. Then lower your legs to the starting position without swinging. Repeat.

Forearms & Neck

Wrist Curl (Barbell)

With your hands about a foot apart, pick up the barbell in the "palms-up" position. Sit on the end of the bench with your feet flat on the floor and about 12-inches apart. Rest your forearms on your thighs so that your wrists extend over your knees about four-inches. Using your wrist, curl the barbell up as high as possible. Pause. Then lower the weight back down as far as possible to the starting position. Repeat. (You can also do wrist curls in the "palms-down" position.)

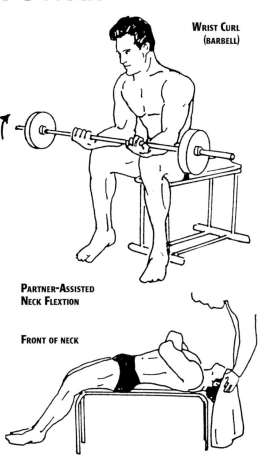

WRIST CURL (BARBELL)

Partner-Assisted Neck Flextion
Front of Neck

To work the front of your neck, lie back on the bench with your head extended over the end. Have your workout partner provide resistance by placing his/her hands on your forehead pushing your head downward in a smooth, even movement as far as you are comfortable. Then your partner gives resistance as you raise your head up and forward (as far as possible) in a smooth, even movement. Repeat.

PARTNER-ASSISTED NECK FLEXTION

FRONT OF NECK

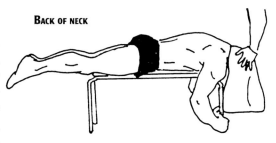

Back of Neck

To work the back of your neck, lie face down on the bench with your head extended over the end. Have your workout partner provide resistance by placing his hands on the back of your head pushing your head downward in a smooth, even movement as far as you are comfortable. Then he gives resistance as you raise your head up and back (as far as possible) in a smooth and even movement. Repeat.

BACK OF NECK

SIDES OF NECK

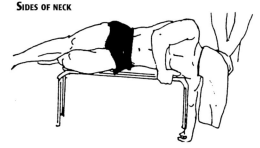

Sides of Neck

The sides of the neck are worked the same as the front and back. The only difference is that you will be on your side on the bench.

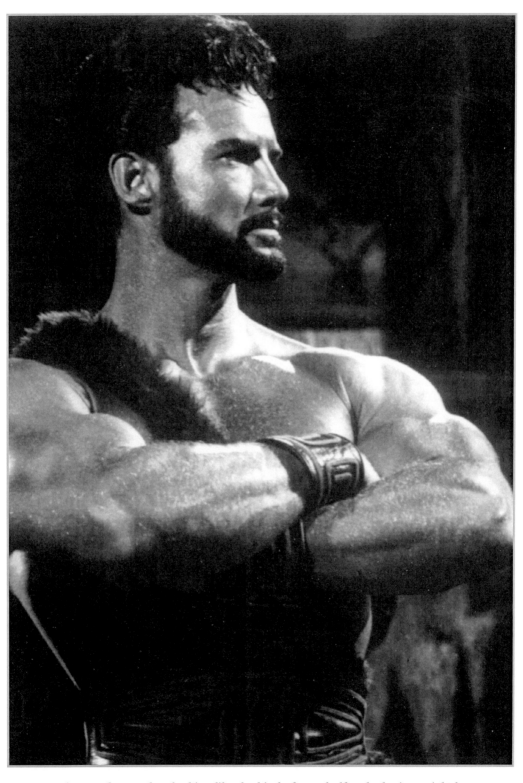

Steve on the set of "Hercules" looking like the kind of man-half-god who just might have gone through some of the adventures in the story.

APPENDIX 3

Steve Reeves' Bodybuilding Principles

1. All muscle groups are to be trained with eight to 12 reps *except calves and abdominals, for which you do 20 reps.*

2. Alternate your repetitions every few months for a couple of weeks to keep your workout from becoming stale. For instance, when you start to get stale on eight to 12 reps, raise your weight and drop down to five to eight reps — or lower your weight and increase your reps to 12 to 15. Do whatever works best for you.

3. Offset your grip on dumbbell flyes and incline curls.

4. Every set should be performed "all-out."

5. Rest just enough in between sets for your partner to perform his/her set.

6. Work your legs last in the workout.

7. Keep your weight the same (or reduce it slightly) with each set.

8. Rest up to three minutes in between training the various body parts.

9. Train no more than three days per week on an alternate-day basis (i.e., Monday, Wednesday, Friday).

10. Train no more than two-and-a-half hours per workout.

11. Drink plenty of water with electrolytes during your workout.

Important Sub-Principles to Remember

1. Always remember that exercising should tire the body but should be relaxing — refreshing to the mind and nervous system; and that to get the most benefit out of an exercise, it is important that you do it correctly.

2. It is important, psychologically, to accomplish small goals that you set for yourself, as it gives a feeling of achievement, and makes you feel like going out and doing more.

3. Balance the difficulty of the exercise with the duration.

4. Keeping fit is like a tire — when used often it keeps inflated; when unused for an extended period of time it gets deflated and requires a lot of exertion to get it inflated again.

5. Start out easy and don't compete against anyone but yourself.

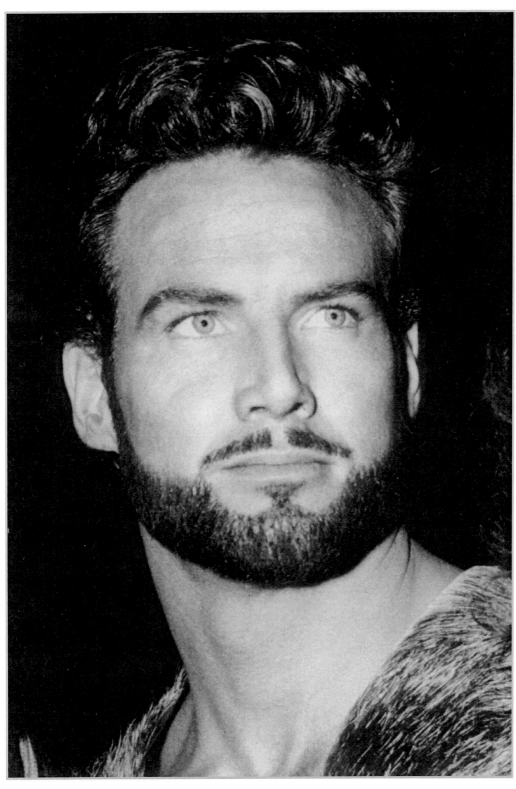

*The look that made him a box office superstar —
"Goliath and the Barbarians" early 1959.*

APPENDIX 4

Awards & Titles Bestowed Upon Steve Reeves

Bodybuilding Titles Won by Steve Reeves

1. Mr. Pacific Coast — Portland, Oregon (1946)
2. Mr. Western America — Los Angeles, California (1947)
3. Mr. America — Chicago, Illinois (1947)
4. Mr. World — Cannes, France (1948)
5. Mr. Universe — London, England (1950)

Bodybuilding and Fitness Awards

1. **The Dan Lurie Award**

    For: "Steve Reeves, World's Greatest Bodybuilder"
    By: W.B.B.G. (World Bodybuilding Guild)
    Location: New York, New York (1973)

2. **World's Greatest Bodybuilder of All Time**

    For: Induction into the "Physical Fitness Hall of Fame"
    By: W.B.B.G. (World Bodybuilding Guild)
    Location: New York, New York (1977)

3. **The World's Most Classic Physique (Gold Sandow Trophy)**

    By: W.A.B.B.A. (World Amateur Bodybuilding Association)
    Location: Paris, France (1977)

4. **World's Most Popular Bodybuilder**

    By: W.A.B.B.A. (World Amateur Bodybuilding Association)
    Location: Madrid, Spain (1977)

5. **Outstanding Contributions to Physical Fitness and Sports**

    By: The President's Council on Physical Fitness and Sports
    Location: New York, New York (1978)

6. **Hall of Fame**

    By: Bodybuilder's Guild — Grand Prix
    Location: Long Beach, California (1981)

7. **Annual Steve Reeves' Award**

    By: The Downtown Athletic Club of New York City
    Location: New York, New York (1981)

8. **Bodybuilding Award of Excellence**

    By: Hall of Fame
    Location: Long Beach, California (1984)

9. **Greatest And Most-Popular Physique Champion of All Time**

    By: The Association of Oldetime Barbell and Strongmen
    Location: New York, New York (1988),

10. **Pioneer of Fitness**

    For: Contributions in promoting physical fitness for all Americans.
    By: The Association of Physical Fitness Centers (1989)

11. **Outstanding Lifetime Achievement and Contributions to the Sport of Bodybuilding**

    By: The Los Angeles Club (1991)

12. Pioneer of Bodybuilding

    By: The Academy of Bodybuilding and Fitness Awards
    Location: Redondo Beach, California (1992)

13. Honorary President of Les Papy's der Muscle 1993

    For: Leadership in Bodybuilding and Fitness
    Location: Ville d'Antibes, France (1993)

14. Movie Legend of the Past

    By: The Academy of Bodybuilding and Fitness Awards
    Location: Redondo Beach, California (1993)

15. Oscar Heidenstam Award

    For: Achievements, sportsmanship, integrity and ambassadorship
    By: NABBA (National Amateur Bodybuilding Association)
    Location: London, England (1994)

16. Pioneer of Bodybuilding and Fitness Award

    By: Gold's Gym, Oakland.
    Location: Oakland, California (1994)

17. Movie Action Hero Award

    By: The Academy of Bodybuilding and Fitness
    Location: Redondo Beach, California (1994)

18. Lifetime Achievement Award

    By: The Academy of Bodybuilding and Fitness
    Location: Redondo Beach, California (1994)

19. Mr. America Lifetime Award

    By: Amateur Athletic Union (AAU)
    Location: Washington, D.C. (1996)

Opposite: On the set of "Morgan the Pirate." Below: "Long Ride from Hell."

Motion Picture Awards Bestowed Upon Steve Reeves

1. Premio Riccione (Most Popular Foreign Actor Award)

   For: Being the most popular foreign actor
   Location: Riccione, Italy (1959)

2. Top Box Office Star

   For: *Hercules* — the undisputed box-office champion of the year.
   By: Box Office (1959)

3. Premio Alio Oro (Golden Wing Award)

   For: Being the number-one box office champion in the world
   By: Italian Cinema
   Location: Chianciano Terme, Italy (1960)

4. Empomeo Ciak

   For: Best Actor in Action Films
   By: The Italian Cinema
   Location: Ischia, Italy (1963)

5. Most Popular Actor in Historic, Biblical and Mythological Films

   Location: Rome, Italy (1964)

6. Silver Boot Award

   By: The Knoxville Western Film Caravan
   Location: Knoxville, Tennessee (1994)

7. Golden Halo Eagle Award

   For: Contributions to the Entertainment Industry and the Performing Arts
   Location: Hollywood, California (1994)

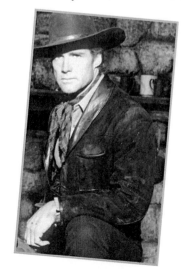

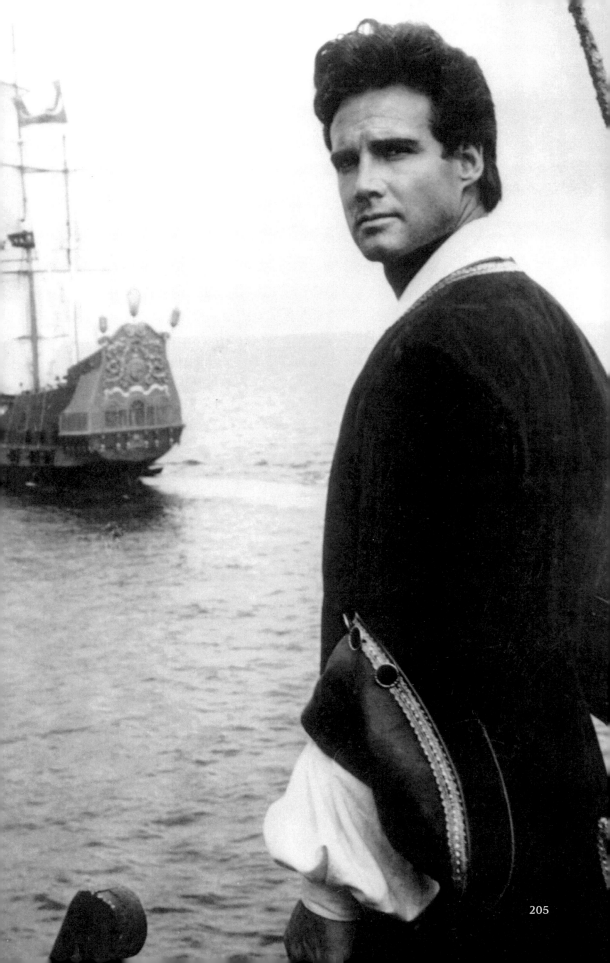

Exercise	Weight	Reps
CLEANS	115	7
PRESS	115	10
CURL	75	15
BENCH CURL	55	15
LEANING ROW	105	10
BENCH PRESS	155	10
SQUAT	200	10
PULL OVER	40	40
BACK BEND	150	30
LATERALS	40	30
UPRIGHT ROW	75	10
FRONT RAISE	30	10
DUMBELL PRESS	75	10
CURL BEHIND NECK	35	15

APPENDIX 5

Bodybuilding's "Holy Grail" -- Steve Reeves' Garage Workout Discovered in April 1994!

by George Helmer

In the November 1994 issue of Flex Magazine, John Little wrote about Steve's first written workout routine that I discovered while in the Oakland, California area. I want to share with you the events leading up to this discovery.

While working as an outside auditor at a client's office in Hayward, California, I began my search. Hayward is located in the South Bay area of San Francisco, approximately five miles south of Oakland. Knowing Steve was reared in Oakland in the 1940s, I began wondering if his house was still standing. If so, it would be great to have a photo of it for the Steve Reeves International Society Newsletter.

Finding the Address

One day after work, I visited the main Oakland library to attempt to locate Steve's old house. The librarian was able to locate the Oakland telephone books from 1939 to 1944. To my amazement, there was his address right in front of my eyes—1477 76th Street, Oakland. I then located the address on a map and drove by to make sure that the house was still there. It was, so the following week I returned with a camera and snapped a few photos of it.

I was going back to Southern California in a few days, so I telephoned Steve and made a luncheon date with him and his wife, Deborah, for the following week. I was anxious to show him a photo of his former home.

We met at a restaurant in Escondido and soon after we ordered our lunch I brought out the photo and asked Steve if it looked familiar. "Why, that's my house in Oakland," remarked Steve, who continued, "I'll tell you an interesting story. I wrote my first workout routine on the inside of the garage wall of that house. I wonder if it's still there." A voice inside me urged me on, "You've got to go back and try to find that workout routine!"

Back in Oakland

The next Monday I was again working in Hayward. A realtor was located across the street from the client's offices, so I stopped by one afternoon and inquired about the property at 1477 76th Street in Oakland. One of the realtors was very helpful and gave me a printout on the property that listed the current owners' names. (This is public information, available in any county where property is recorded.)

That same day I sent a letter to the owners of the property, telling them about the workout routine that was written inside of their garage, and asked permission to come and see if it was still there. To my surprise, the next day I received a telephone call from Mrs. Gloria Hartman, one of the owners. She said I could come over and look for the routine in the garage.

I telephoned Steve that night and told him about my contact with Mrs. Hartman, and that she gave me permission to look for the routine. I asked if he remembered where it was located. He said that it was about three feet in on the right side of the garage wall, halfway up, in between the stud 2x4s on the wood siding. I telephoned Mrs. Hartman and arranged to drop by in a couple of days.

Hot on the Trail

I arrived at the Hartman's late one afternoon. Mrs. Hartman led me to the garage at the rear of the property and opened the door. As soon as I saw the inside walls, I knew I had a problem. The walls had been drywalled many years ago, judging from the looks of it.

I asked Mrs. Hartman, "If I replaced the drywall, can I cut out one section?" To my continued surprise she agreed. Since I did not have any tools with me, I made arrangements to return with tools on Saturday morning.

That Saturday turned out to be an enormous emotional roller coaster. I couldn't wait to open the wall and find that routine. Using a tape measure, I marked off the spot where it was supposed to be. Next, I had to remove a cabinet from the wall before proceeding to cut through the drywall. Finally, the drywall was down and so were my spirits—no routine was there. Mrs. Hartman said maybe it was elsewhere on the wall, and to move down the wall a bit. I did and still turned up nothing.

Then I noticed the garage looked as if it had been remodeled and added on to at some time in the past. I thought maybe the routine was located in the

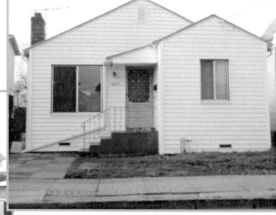

The Oakland home where the teenage Reeves began his bodybuilding regime and the garage that was his gym.

Steve's routine revealed to present owners, Mr. and Mrs. Hartman.

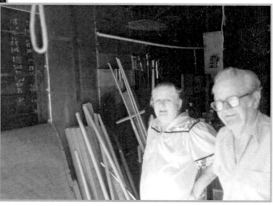

added-on section. Mrs. Hartman gave me her "O.K." to check in the back section. Again,. I took off move drywall and faced another disappointment. No routine.

I was ready to give up, and told Mrs. Hartman that there was a good chance it either was removed long ago, or it was somewhere else in the garage. I told her I did not want to remove any more drywall from the garage. I was ready to quit, but she wasn't. She suggested I try the wall opposite my first try. I was hesitant to cut up any more walls in that garage, but thought I would give it one more try.

I very carefully cut and removed another piece of drywall. It was backed by tar paper, which I also carefully cut. As I took a hold of the top edge of the tar paper and began pulling down, I saw some writing! My heart started pounding and I knew this was it! There, hidden for years, was Steve's original routine, fifteen exercises with the amount of reps and weight used for each!

At that point I told Mrs. Hartman that the person who wrote it all down was none other than Steve Reeves, world-famous bodybuilder and actor. She doubted me until I brought out the documentation I brought along to show her. I purchased that piece of garage wall from her and now Steve's very first handwritten routine is preserved and in our possession.

By the way, I am out of the drywall business forever!

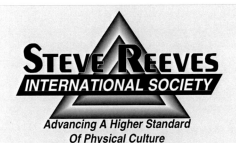

Advancing A Higher Standard Of Physical Culture

Become a Member of the Steve Reeves International Society

We are excited at the adventure we have embarked upon with the help of Steve Reeves. We have many plans for the future, and want you to participate in these endeavors with us. The organization was founded by George Helmer, with the express approval of Steve Reeves. The Steve Reeves International Society promotes well-being, both physically and mentally. We are committed to ensure that Steve's integrity and image are never compromised. The Society is totally dedicated to this living legend.

We have been publishing a very exciting and informative quarterly newsletter since January 1995. Each newsletter contains 16-pages of great stories and valuable information, including articles on Steve's training and nutritional practices, and a continuing series of biographical pieces on Steve Reeve's life.

You are given a wonderful, in-depth look into his movies and the world that surrounded them. There are news briefs and a classified ad section where you can buy and sell Steve Reeves collectibles! We offer special limited-edition (collector) items, plus great-looking T-shirts, beverage mugs, videos, Reeves calendars and much more.

Get your one-year newsletter subscription and lifetime membership in the Steve Reeves International Society for only $25.00. Send a check or money order to:

> Steve Reeves International Society
> P. O. Box 2625
> Malibu, California 90265
> (626) 287-9128

Steve Reeves Photographs

Here is your chance to get a personally autographed photo of Steve Reeves.

You can choose from either (a) movie, (b) bodybuilding, or any combination of the two categories. For photo prices and selection sample sheet, write to:

> Steve Reeves Classic Image Enterprises
> P. O. Box 807
> Valley Center, California 92082

Also, check out *Steve Reeves* on the web.

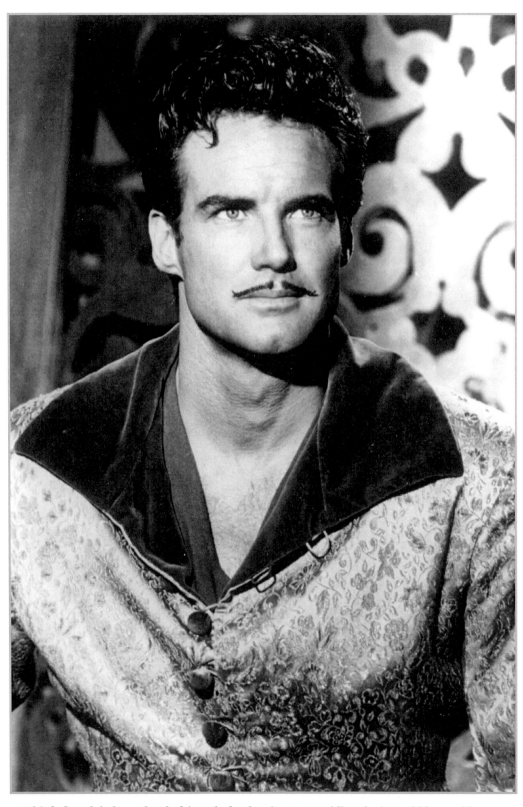

"Thief of Baghdad"— a lovely fairy tale for the cinema providing the intrepid hero with many chances to show off his strength and stamina.

APPENDIX 6

What the Press Said about Steve Reeves

"The biggest crowd ever assembled in Los Angeles for a physical-culture show applauded, cheered and gasped whenever STEVE REEVES posed during the selection of 'Mr. Pacific Coast'....Steve out-glowed, outshone, and out-muscled the competition. This kid is sensational...he hasn't a single weak spot in his make-up...quick as a cat in movement, dramatic, enthusiastic, a natural showman, and vivacious as a powerful youth could ever be...and with a vibrating happy personality that fairly radiates tremendous vitality and force....It was quite a sight to see him hold all his trophies in his arms. I doubt if anyone else has ever won so many at one show. It is difficult to impart with words exactly how he looked while he posed. He turned from one display to another, but every one of the many thousands of eyes glued to the mass of muscles under excellent lighting blinked an eye I am sure. He seemed out of this world, just as though a superman had suddenly appeared on the pedestal...a great kid who is going to win more and more cups and trophies and whose fabulous physique will spread to all parts of the world. Mark this prophecy. I will not be wrong in my prediction, and I am daring to make this statement....There isn't one athlete in the country who is not applauding Steve...He deserves every thing that may come his way....He stands but one step away from the 'Mr. America' title..."

— Walter Marcyan, **Your Physique**, August 1947

"It is unbelievable that anyone could have such huge muscular size and yet retain the perfect balance in proportions and the excellent muscle separation that STEVE REEVES displayed at the 1947 Mr. America contest....We have never seen a man who looked finer in his street or dress clothes."

— Peary Rader, **Iron Man**, July 1947

"I am sure if one of the Ancient Greeks came to life today and saw our new 'Mr. America,' STEVE REEVES, he would find it hard to believe that Steve was not a reincarnation of the body of one of those superior beings from Mount Olympus. There are great things ahead for this boy, and I can see him following the star-dust trail to Mount Olympus!"

— Lou Hanagan, **Your Physique**, July 1947

"STEVE REEVES' first radio appearance came a day after he had won his title...He appeared on ABC's coast-to-coast network show, 'Ladies be Seated,' as a guest of Johnny Olson. Before a packed studio audience and millions of radio listeners, Steve explained how he obtained his title-winning physique. Our reporter tells us that radio tubes all over the country melted with the broadcast sighs and exclamations of the radio audience when Steve revealed his magnificent torso... Steve was also a guest of Nate Gross, Chicago's noted rancher and news columnist, at his famous High Dresser Ranch at the Blackstone Hotel. Nate, a man who numbers celebrities and movie stars by dozens among his close friends, affirms that Steve will be a natural for a movie hero....'He's got everything it takes!'....Hundreds of letters concerning Steve have been pouring into the office, with requests for his photographs mounting daily....We predict that Steve will take an all-time high place among the 'Mr. Americas.'"

— Abe Marmel, **Bodybuilder**, August 1947

"A thunderous approbation of hand clapping that gave way to cheers and whistles from the audience let the judges know in no uncertain terms their acceptance of REEVES as 'Mr. America.' You have to see this young man to really appreciate his build and good looks. Photos don't do him justice; he's twice as good as his pictures. It would be utter futility for me to try to describe in mere words his physique...'breath-taking' might give you some idea of the audience reaction....As readers will recall, I never did lean heavily to 'Mr. America' contests when these contests were in their embryonic stages. It was my contention that such shows were not for the real 'iron man.' Now I've changed my opinion!...I believe a change has been wrought in the conception of the perfect male physique...Now we have the new streamlined conception of the perfect masculine physique and Steve Reeves epitomizes that conception. His tremendous breadth of shoulders and extreme sliminess of waist are symbolic of the new physique. He exemplifies speed and grace rather than brute strength.... I sincerely believe that if the immortal Sandow could have been called back from the Land of Shades to step upon the posing platform against Reeves, he would have lost!"

— Gordon Venables, **Strength & Health**, August 1947

"I was the first person to interview STEVE REEVES after he won the coveted 'Mr. America' title. He had just stepped off the stage and was still holding the huge gold trophy. Seeing him in his bathing trunks, a perfect physical specimen, like all women I wondered how he would look in a suit. Taking in his broad shoulders and brown hair, I decided I would like him best in a brown English tweed. Or should it be a tuxedo? I was having a hard time making up my mind. My imagination went a little further as I believe all gals who meet Steve Reeves will dream, and I thought of him as a Saturday night date. He filled the bill perfectly. I snapped out of my reverie when our photographer unceremoniously pushed me toward STEVE and said, 'Get in the picture!' Don't get me wrong; I didn't mind. And don't think I get dreamy eyed over every male I interview, but you just can't help liking Steve Reeves..."

— Valerie Zawila, **Bodybuilder Magazine**, December 1947

"STEVE REEVES recently took his movie test in New York City at Columbia Studios. One expert critic said: 'The man is sensational...when he smiles, the whole screen lights up. He even looks more muscular on screen than off, and makes most movie stars look weak beside him. All he needs is a break and he is sure to go places.'..."

— **Muscle Power**, June 1948

"New York photographer Gebbe recently said: I have seen all the 'Mr. Americas,' but REEVES tops them all...I doubt if there will ever be another 'Mr. America' like him!"

— **Muscle Power**, June 1948

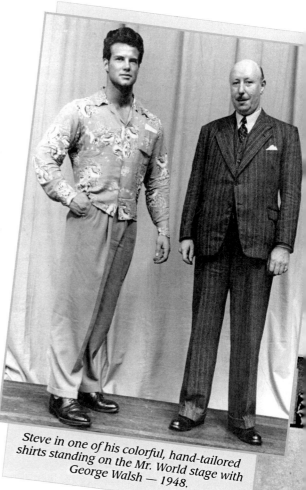

Steve in one of his colorful, hand-tailored shirts standing on the Mr. World stage with George Walsh — 1948.

"Steve Reeves and I were walking down Broadway the other night. It was quite an experience. Every beautiful gal we passed turned to take another look. Several stopped to ask for autographs thinking for sure he must be some great movie star. One woman driving past in a car almost piled up into the back of another car. She was looking at Steve and not at the road in front of her. We walked into a restaurant and two smart fellows with two good looking girls joked in stage whispers: Watch the shoulders come off when he takes his coat off...did you ever see such padding! He must have a couple of pillows stuffed in there!' Steve smiled, the girls blushed with embarrassment, and the men scowled with scorn. Steve took off his coat to hang it up and four pairs of eyes almost popped out of four different heads. I couldn't help thinking what a jolt those people would have got if Steve had stripped to the waist!"

— **Muscle Power,** June 1948

"STEVE REEVES, tops among the greatest, is presently completing his film training in Hollywood..."

— **Your Physique**, June 1948

"While the judges' results were undergoing a final tally at the 1948 'Canada's Most Perfect Physique Contest,' the star attraction was presented — STEVE REEVES — and what an ovation he was given...Every newspaper in Montreal, both French and English, ran photos and write-ups on Steve..."

— **Your Physique**, February 1948

"Magnificently developed STEVE REEVES is now in London and will compete in the 'Mr. Universe' contest at the Scala Theater on August 13..."

— **Vigour**, August 1948

"A spectator at the 1948 AAU 'Mr. America,' STEVE REEVES was called up from his seat among the audience. Gladly he consented to pose. Then Clarence Ross was spotted and went up on stage. Voices demanded a posing contest....George Wilcut called for a pair of posing trunks and the battle was on. Reeves went on first and gave muscular displays amid thunderous applause, and his posing was filled with determination. Ross followed with his usual tranquil style. Both looked great and I think I am forced to call it a draw. Anyway, I'll save my neck by stating so!"

— **Muscle Power,** September 1948

"STEVE REEVES' brief posing routine at the 1948 AAU 'Mr. America' held everyone spellbound. Steve looked wonderful — better than ever! ... An amusing episode took place backstage. Mighty Mac Batchelor challenged Steve to punch him full-force in the abdomen. Steve did it! And believe it or not, big Mac never budged from this severe blow."

— **Muscle Power,** August 1948

"The gang at Bert Goodrich's gym, where STEVE REEVES is now working-out, stands at full attention while Steve trains. What a back that kid has..from here to here!"

— **Muscle Power,** August 1948

"Without a doubt, STEVE REEVES has one of the finest developed bodies ever seen anywhere or any time in history!"

— **Iron Man**, September 1948

"The big class of men of six-feet and over gave the crowd at the 1948 'Mr. Universe' its first sight of STEVE REEVES. There was a demonstration of enthusiasm and the audience gave him a terrific reception. Steve has a super build and the international throng that watched him was not at all slow to show their appreciation."

— **Strength & Health**, October 1948

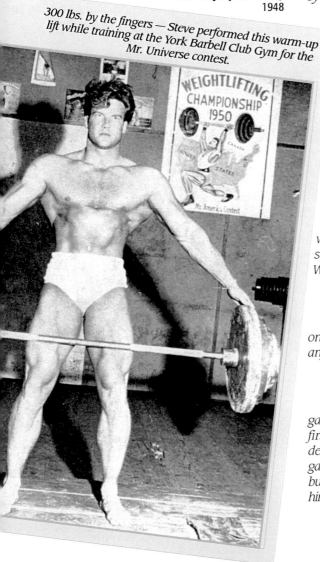

300 lbs. by the fingers — Steve performed this warm-up lift while training at the York Barbell Club Gym for the Mr. Universe contest.

"STEVE REEVES the great!....gave an exhibition posing routine during the 1948 'Mr. Pacific Coast' contest. He caused excitement among the entire audience and was called back for an encore."

— **Muscle Power**, November 1948

"As this is being written, Armand Tanny, Bert Goodrich, STEVE REEVES, and others are peacefully sailing upon the cerulean-blue Pacific for a day or two."

— **Muscle Power**, December 1948

"During our first few days at the beach, onlookers got a good look at Steve Reeves as an athlete. Any movement of his body was dazzling. When his powerful legs churned up a cloud of sand in a flat-out sprint, we saw the most efficiently graceful running machine since Man-O-War."

-– Armand Tanny, **Muscle Power**, 1948

"STEVE REEVES and Armand Tanny both recently cleaned 220 pounds from the kneeling position. Try it yourself sometime!"

— **Muscle Power**, December 1948

"The magnificent STEVE REEVES was next. This man has the most marvelous arms and shoulders. His legs are terrifically developed. He never fails to be a sensation whenever he comes on the stage."

— **Iron Man**, April 1949

"The January cover of STEVE REEVES which appeared on Your Physique, has created more comments in the history of our publication than any other."

— **Muscle Power**, May 1949

"STEVE REEVES now in the greatest condition of his career....It was a privilege to watch him pose at Muscle Beach. Wait until you see some of his latest pictures. You'll be amazed!"

— **Muscle Power**, February 1949

"STEVE REEVES has flown to Hawaii for two weeks of posing and relaxation....He's really cashing in on his muscles."

— **Muscle Power**, September 1949

"STEVE REEVES, strolling around looking in great shape, despite the fact — as he tells me — that he has not done a bit of training for over four months."

— **Muscle Power**, September 1949

"STEVE REEVES, at present writing, is doing his stuff again down in Mexico City. Sure hops around!"

— **Muscle Power**, January 1949

"STEVE REEVES back once more at Muscle Beach from his flight from Mexico City. He was dressed this time in a natty blue-gray suit with a bright-blue tie and a blue pocket handkerchief. I pounced on him and asked 'Habla Usted Espanol?' 'No Earle,' Steve replied, 'I only learned two words of Spanish... 'Si Senorita!' '"

— **Muscle Power**, December 1949

"Flash! STEVE REEVES just bought an electric juicer to pulverize all the vegetables, egg shells, greens, etc."

— **Muscle Power**, May 1949

"STEVE REEVES does hardly any training anymore. He wants to lose some of his muscles as he had too much for a motion-picture contract. Steve wants to get down to 190."

— **Muscle Power**, June 1949

"STEVE REEVES returned to Hollywood from nowhere — or from wherever he was and brought with him a brand-new upper-lip decoration. He is now assistant instructor to Bert Goodrich at the latter's gym. And Steve still wears those loud handmade shirts. And he's in grand condition, too!"

— **Muscle Power**, July 1949

"STEVE REEVES, back in Hollywood again with his unusual sport shirts. Only Steve can wear 'em!"

— Muscle Power, March 1950

"Along the boulevard, STEVE REEVES seen lurching in and out of crowds with long strides while making the rounds of men's furnishing stores."

— Muscle Power, May 1950

"Final Flash! STEVE REEVES now running up and down the Hollywood hills reducing his weight because of a motion-picture contract which requires he get under 200 lbs."

— **Muscle Power**, June 1950

"STEVE REEVES is one of the greatest physical culturists of all time. No other man has had such a fabulous development."

— **Iron Man**, January 1950

"A popular victory was scored by STEVE REEVES in the 1950 'Mr. Universe' contest in London on the 24th of June."

— **Strength & Health**, August 1950

"STEVE REEVES, physical-culture's Apollo of Popularity. For the many readers who have written for his address, it is..."

— **Health Review**, November 1950

"Since Reg Park and STEVE REEVES are both about the same height and bodyweight and very impressive when clothed - Reg was stopped going through customs with the question: 'Are you 'Mr. America, Steve Reeves?' Walking on Broadway, Reg was stopped numerous times during a stroll by people who asked him if he was Reeves. Reg got tired shaking his head no, but was mighty impressed with the popularity of Steve Reeves in New York City. Wait until Reg gets out to the West Coast. He'll have to wear a sign reading: 'No, I am not Steve Reeves! I am Reg Park of Britain!'"

— **Muscle Power**, May 1950

"Enough water to make a pond was sweated out of STEVE REEVES during the several weeks he was here at York training arduously for the 'Mr. Universe' contest."

— **Strength & Health**, August 1950

"STEVE REEVES, in case you're interested, is now in New York City filming a TV engagement which plans to run a long serial of connecting episodes featuring Reeves."

— **Muscle Power**, February 1951

"Notice how STEVE REEVES resembles Li'l Abner? He's sure to be a hit in a movie version. Maybe we ought to start a campaign for him."

— **Muscle Power**, April 1951

"When STEVE REEVES won the 'Mr. America' in 1947, to my mind he was superb. The man had everything ....There was the physique of the century...a wonderful God-given combination of grace, power, size, and definition."

— Reg Park, **Your Physique**, July 1951

"Almost daily, TV viewers have the opportunity to see STEVE REEVES on the Ralph Edwards NBC television show."

— **Strength & Health**, August 1952

"Bodybuilders from Muscle Beach

thoroughly dominated the program of the three-day Beach Festival held over the Labor Day weekend at Santa Monica. In the tug-of-war, the big highlight of the first day's program, the Muscle Beach contingent could find no competition, so STEVE REEVES and George Eifferman were delegated to choose-up sides for an all-Muscle Beach tug-of-war exhibition. After a three-minute pull, Reeves and company had gained about 6 inches to win the first bout."

— **Muscle Power**, February 1952

"Rumor has it that STEVE REEVES is now down to 187 pounds. This great loss in weight was made by demand of Steve's movie bosses."

— **Muscle Power**, March 1952

"STEVE REEVES, the perfect interpretation of the Theseus type of physique, has a handsomeness of features unsurpassed to this day. He will always be in a class by himself, for his development — in its beauty - is admired by people of widely varying tastes, types and classes."

— **Mr. Universe**, March 1952

"STEVE REEVES, according to reports, has just signed another 36 week contract with the Ralph Edwards Show."

— **Muscle Power**, November 1952

"STEVE REEVES, looking slimmer, tells me he weighs 195 pounds. But somehow or other, I think everyone misses the huge muscles he had around the time he became 'Mr. Universe.'"

— **Muscle Power**, August 1953

"REEVES is THE NAME! He will always be thought of as one of the world's greatest greats."

— **Health & Strength**, October 1953

"At the present time STEVE REEVES is appearing in the successful 'Kismet' musical on Broadway."

— **Strength & Health**, July 1954

"In a moment of weakness the other night, I turned on the TV set to Steve Allen's 'Tonight' program, and was agreeably surprised by the guest appearance of STEVE REEVES, an exponent of weight training. This TV appearance served to confirm the fact that Steve is somewhat less lumpy than in days of yore....It all adds up to one conclusion. Would you rather have lumps of muscle or hunks of currency? Personally I think his TV appearance on a very popular program will sell more barbells than any of his former appearances as an avowed muscleman at the various physique shows. The public taste is for moderation in physical size."

— Harry Paschall, **Strength & Health**, April 1955

"I have not seen a new picture of STEVE REEVES posing in a long time. Doesn't he pose anymore? He still maintains good form but his muscle-size has lessened somewhat. It is natural that he refrains from posing under these circumstances."

— **Muscle Power**, November 1955

"STEVE REEVES is the idol of almost every kid that takes up bodybuilding. In fact, he is the reason they take it up!"

— **Vim**, April 1956

"STEVE REEVES is the great American yardstick against whose magnificent manhood all athletes are measured... All of us owe a great debt to Steve. He is a champion's champion!"

— **Adonis**, April 1956

"STEVE REEVES, the world's best built

man, has just opened a fine gym in Miami Beach, Florida."

— **Iron Man**, May 1956

"Despite STEVE REEVES' frequent absences from the game, his popularity from the time he first wore the 'Mr. America' crown, up to the present, has never waned. A restless, sometimes impatient, and often impulsive individual, he lives for the present and insists that it treats him well. To bodybuilders, he is commonly known as 'Mr. Everything' Tall, handsome, massively-muscled with a bon vivant outlook, he is a man of ideals, nonetheless, and a man of firm ideas. Add a tenacity of purpose and a refusal to admit defeat, and you have a smattering of the complexity that has become loved as Steve Reeves."

— **Muscle Builder**, November 1956

"Mickey Hagarty is now in Hollywood and can often be seen training with STEVE REEVES."

— **Muscle Power**, August 1957

"STEVE REEVES is now sporting a beard. Makes him look like an Italian aristocrat — or something."

— **Muscle Power**, August 1957

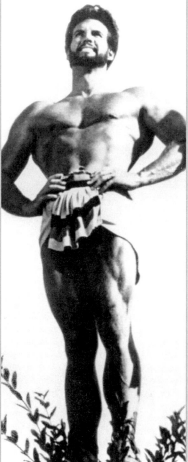

"That well-trimmed looking beard that STEVE REEVES sported, which gave him added dignity in appearance, had to be suddenly shaved off. Steve received a hurry call from the studios to play a part in two TV shows and when he walked in to work, the first words he heard were: 'Off with the chin-grass!' Steve, who had carefully raised the facial crop for a motion-picture in Italy, began growing the whiskers all over again, for he flies to Rome in a few days."

— **Muscle Power**, December 1957

"Many of you have asked about STEVE REEVES. He is now in Italy starting in a movie over there where Steve is a great hero to the people."

— **Iron Man**, September 1957

"The adoration of the male physique that characterized the grandeur of Greece and Rome is being rekindled in modern Italy by one lone American, STEVE REEVES! 'Mr. America,' 'Mr. World, 'Mr. Universe, or as we frequently call him — 'Mr. Everything' — has become a national hero."

— **Mr. America**, August 1958

"STEVE REEVES is back in the States after spending a year in Italy, He bought a ranch and intends to raise horses and avocados. Maybe my ears heard wrongly and perhaps he said 'horses and flies,' as these usually go together."

— **Muscle Builder**, July 1958

"Mario Lanza thinks nothing of telephoning from overseas to his parents and friends in the U.S. His latest call came from London to Terry Robinson. He asked Terry lots of questions, and inquired of STEVE REEVES."

— **Muscle Builder**, July 1958

"On screen or off, STEVE REEVES demonstrates the rewards in store for muscular lads who exercise regularly."

— **Life**, August 1959

" 'Hercules,' starring STEVE REEVES, has shattered every box office record in its initial saturation engagements throughout New England."

— **Box Office**, August 1959

"Heavy overall promotion resulted in amazing box office grosses for 'Hercules' in the downtown Milwaukee theaters."

— **Box Office**, August 1959

" 'Hercules' showed the greatest box office strength in Cleveland, piling up a tremendous 210 percent rating."

— **Box Office**, August 1959

"Indianapolis teenagers are high on STEVE REEVES as 'Hercules.' It set the pace with heavy attendance over the weekend."

— **Box Office**, August 1959

"On the infrequent days when he is not working, STEVE REEVES leaves his apartment in the American Palace Hotel at noon and shoulders his way through a horde of youthful admirers. He goes directly to Doney's on the Via Veneto, there to sit at a sidewalk table until dinner time drinking orange juice and signing autographs for the unending line of respectful fans who have anticipated his appearance. Many of the teenage boys have copied Steve's beard, and all of them refer to him affectionately as 'Ercole.' "

— Embassy Pictures Publicity Release, April 1959

"As this is being written, a Manila newspaper has arrived and 'Hercules' is making a sensation at Manila's Odeon Theater."

— **Muscle Builder**, June 1959

"Eastern movie moguls have got their spies out looking for a bodybuilder built along Tarzan lines. The specifications? 'Give us someone like Reeves...you know, tall, dark, massively built, with an extraordinarily handsome face, perfect teeth, 18-inch arms, 29-inch waist, and a 50-inch chest.' We dutifully explained that a Reeves comes along once in a lifetime. Afraid they're gonna' have to take someone a little less 'god-like,' or Reeves-like!"

— **Muscle Builder**, October 1959

"Muscles — like WOW! ...Barbells, pulleys,

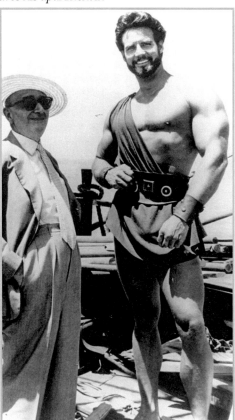

and weights have made STEVE REEVES the giant of a man he is today....Montana born Steve was picked to play 'Hercules' because the Italian producers believe his is the most beautiful body in the world!"

— **Movie Mirror**, October 1959

" 'Goliath and the Barbarians' in its American premiere engagement at the Roosevelt Theater in Chicago, broke the 30 year-old house record for Thanksgiving day business."

— **Box Office**, December 1959

"I was three weeks in tracking down stalwart STEVE REEVES for an interview. He was cruising in the Greek islands and when I finally got word to him that I wanted to talk to him he came back to Rome a week early from his vacation. Our trans-Atlantic connection was so clear he sounded as if he were in the next room. The first thing Steve told me was that he would see me in the middle of February, when he would be in Hollywood and would like to drop by my house for a glass of tomato juice or ginger ale, and I told him I was looking forward to meeting him. 'What are you doing in the Greek islands?' I asked. Steve laughed and said, 'I've made so many pictures of ancient Greece, I wanted to see what it was all about. I was greatly impressed, and loved Athens. I think it's very much like Majorca and its surrounding islands which are so beautiful.' I agreed with him on the beauty of Majorca, where I spent two weeks in 1956. Because of his outstanding physique, Steve has won many 'Mr.' contests. . . 'How do you keep in such good shape?' I asked. 'I've always been an athlete and played football in school.' Steve said. 'I ride horseback and do a lot of swimming. Since I've been in Italy I've taken up underwater fishing, which is a great sport here.' Realizing we would soon own the telephone company if we talked much longer, I thought I'd better ask him about the romance department. 'I have no special romances,' said the handsome hero, just the usual dates. I don't want to get married for at least two years. I am so grateful for the way my pictures are going. I want to pursue my career further, and give it every chance to build up before I get married."

— **Louella Parsons**, **Los Angeles Herald Examiner**, January 24, 1960

"The popularity of STEVE REEVES continues to grow. Steve is the top star in Europe, and becoming more popular in the USA. 'Goliath and the Barbarians,' Steve's latest, is playing to SRO audiences in NYC."

— **Iron Man**, April 1960

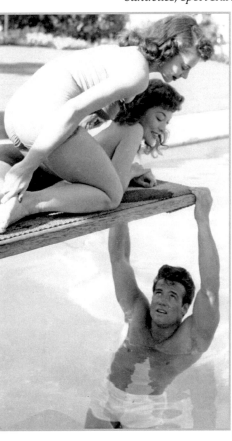

"Shake the male dreams of both Mae West and Jayne Mansfield together, add the spice of youth and you have STEVE REEVES, the 'build' to end them all! ... At the moment he is piling up a fortune as producer Joseph E. Levine's hero rounding up the legendary Greek musclemen in sequences that have ravished literature but lined both their cloaks with a permanent golden fleece....Reeves' muscles bulge like money, but Steve has a word of caution on wine, women, and weight,....'I make sure I get ten hours of sleep, drink good clean water, and keep my mind on horses when it comes to beauty.' This cowpoke rustles books. Steve has a little Italian number he calls his 'occasional.' We saw her. Pony tail or no, she's no horse!"

— **Spencer Hardy**, **King Features Syndicate**, April 1960

"It's REEVES month again! Every columnist from Louella Parsons to Hedda Hopper is chronicling his every move. We've heard a rumor that the US mint is working on a split-shift, trying to coin enough money for this magnificent man who has turned his muscles into moneybags."

— **Muscle Builder**, July 1960

"STEVE REEVES is now earning $200,000 a picture, and he is presently seen on almost as many marketable products as Mickey Mouse....'Hercules' comic books, games, statuettes, sport shirts, bathing trunks, etc..."

— Sidney Skolsky, **Hollywood Citizen News**, July 21, 1960

"Compared with some of the Americans already in Rome, the athletes arriving for the Olympics last week looked like a bunch of scrawny adolescents. It was a good bet that none of them had ever withstood the pull of two horses going in opposite directions, or bare-handedly saved Christians from lions, or even fought a giant crab under water. But over at Rome's Titanus studios, STEVE REEVES had done or was doing all these things...Reeves told Newsweek in Rome last week: 'I can put on 20 pounds of muscle in two weeks, or I can take it off. For this role, 190 — which I am now — is about right. Too many muscles can get in your way. You've got to have enough to get people interested, but not so much that you scare them off."

— **Newsweek**, August 29, 1960

"As handsome a hunk of man as ever adorned a beach — or elsewhere - is STEVE REEVES... Steve is patient with autograph seekers, but he gets a little annoyed at women who reach out to feel his biceps. 'It gets pretty tiresome' he says. 'They don't even ask my permission..... 'Worst of all' - he says - 'is the funny look some women get in their eyes. I don't quite know what they're thinking.' Don't worry about it, Stevie boy, just take good care of those muscles and hurry home!"

— May Okon, **New York Sunday News**, June 26, 1960

"Upon the completion of the Academy Award winning film, Ben-Hur, STEVE REEVES purchased the Andalusian stallion used in the film as a gift for his folks."

— **Movie Mirror**, December 1960

"STEVE REEVES is a traveler. At home, you'll have him to yourself; overseas he'll be mobbed everywhere, Meet him on 'ladies' day' at the gym where he works out and you'll find him gentler than those muscles lead you to believe."

— **Hollywood Secrets Annual**, 1960

"The star who had the greatest impact in movie theaters last year is a heroically-muscled Titan named STEVE REEVES. Steve has caused female hearts to flutter all around the world."

— **Hollywood Secrets Yearbook**, 1960

"One by one, the big limousines pulled up in front of Milari's plush Theater Rudulfo for the world premiere of the widely ballyhooed movie, 'Hercules Unchained.' Lining both sides of the theater, a crowd of women was held in check by two rows of carabinierri When a big Mercedes pulled up and a brawny, broad-shouldered, bearded male stepped out, a full-throated roar rose from the crowd. The carabinierri braced themselves against the wave of screaming, hysterical women. Then the surging women broke their ranks and swarmed over their hero in an orgy of adulation. Before the carabinierri could reform into a flying wedge that bulldozed through the crowd, STEVE REEVES' jacket and shirt were ripped off his back and his naked arms and shoulders were covered with tiny scarlet imprints of no less than 75 amorous lips ...If Steve Reeves isn't the biggest thing in show business, he certainly is the hottest! 'It's the girls,' says one prominent Hollywood producer. 'They're wild about him. He has become a universal sex-symbol, a kind of male Marilyn Monroe....It figures,' says showman Levine. 'They scour the world for girls with gorgeous bodies — and men love them. What about the girls? Why not give them something? Especially since women outnumber men and make up the bulk of the movie-going public.'. . . Levine's shrewd hunch paid off handsomely. Today, a battery of 20 secretaries barely keeps up with the avalanche of 5,000 letters a day Steve Reeves gets from amorous fans. Many of them are headily uninhibited and cannot be reprinted in a magazine....Many of his fans are older, married women who see in the heavily-muscled Reeves a personification of virile masculinity. Psychiatrists view his popularity as an expression of women's deep-seated yearning to be dominated... 'It is basically a healthy expression,' says one prominent psychiatrist. 'Women are getting tired of dominating men. They want to be feminine, to express their basic natures. When they see Reeves, they imagine themselves succumbing to this lordly male.' For whatever reasons, the girls flock to his movies. Record crowds greet his epics all over America. One manager complained that he had to change his lobby display, featuring a life-size cut of Steve Reeves, three times a day. 'Every couple of hours' he said, 'the picture would be unrecognizable - completely covered with lipstick prints. And I mean <u>completely</u> covered... Reeves is probably the only matinee idol in history

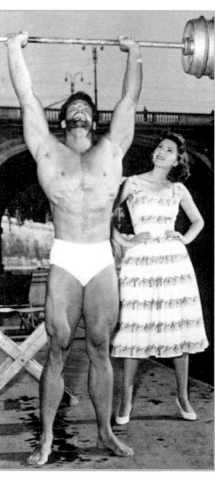

whose torso is better known than his face. Recently, he spent an afternoon at an Italian Riviera resort town. Fully clothed, he strolled about the town undisturbed. Then he stripped to go for a swim. As soon as he appeared in his bathing trunks he was spotted. A mob of women took after him and Steve had to sprint to the local jailhouse for safety. Now, Hollywood bigwigs are wondering whether this popularity is just a fluke, a passing fad? 'He'll last as long as women like real he-men,' says one knowing Hollywood agent, 'and I don't see that changing for a long, long time!'"

— John Ginfreddi, **Scene**, October 1960

"One of the most powerful stars today is a fellow named STEVE REEVES. He went to Europe and became a smash. Every allowable inch of Reeves body has been shown here and all over the world."

— Bill Slocum, **Boston Daily Record**, June 22, 1961

"STEVE REEVES, currently in 'Thief of Baghdad,' I will marry again, live in Rome, make more epics."

— **Teen Stars Album**, 1961

"The Perry Como Show, the number one program in the musical variety field, used a gigantic enlargement of the February cover of our magazine, featuring STEVE REEVES on the cover, as the center theme of a display of the nation's leading magazines."

— **Tomorrow's Man**, March 1961

"We get all kinds of crazy letters about STEVE REEVES. But one of the oldest was from some bodybuilder in the wilds of Arkansas who wrote: 'I am a fan of Steve Reeves. I saw 'Hercules' four times a day for a whole week. I went in the theater at 1:00 p.m. and stayed right through till the last feature was over at 11:00 p.m. Now I hear Steve is sick with some rear (sic!) disease ...' Undoubtedly this fan meant 'rare' disease, but Steve is bursting with good health."

— **Muscle Builder**, November 1961

"STEVE REEVES is not ill...he does not have a rare disease...he has not fallen on the set and broken his back...he is not broke...he is not falling apart...and he still has all 32 dazzling while teeth (the better to snap at his critics, ya' know!) and he is rolling in money. We're now receiving about 300 letters each week from worried bodybuilders, so we want to set your minds at ease."

— **Muscle Builder**, November 1961

"The ultimate in physical perfection was on display at the 1950 'Mr. Universe' contest. STEVE REEVES the incomparable! Will we ever see such muscular perfection again"

— **Mr. America**, June 1962

'This issue is inscribed to that greatest of physique stars, STEVE REEVES. Every day we receive hundreds of letters from all over the globe asking for his exact training routine, his photograph, his autograph, or news of him and his screen activities. His appeal is elemental and universal... He is at once lodestar and pied piper. The most undeveloped young men everywhere are magnetically drawn to him, are inspired by him, and in their dreams each night every Walter Mitty is Steve Reeves with the world as his oyster."

— **Demi-Gods**, September 1962

"STEVE REEVES bought a huge ranch in Oregon for his mother and stepfather. He wanted to get them away from the smog and smoke of Southern California. Steve flew back to Rome shortly after getting them located and is now making another film."

— **Muscle Builder**, October 1962

"Reports are that STEVE REEVES looks just like he did when he won the Mr. America in 1947... if Steve has found the fountain of youth, we wish he would work us in on the deal."

— **Muscle Builder**, December 1962

"STEVE REEVES was seen in Cairo's Nile Hilton Hotel gym ... His physique is just as Great as it was when he won the 'Mr. America' contest!"

— **Muscle Builder**, March 1963

"A perfect body without a certain perfection of mind is slipping back to the extinct giants that roamed the earth' says STEVE REEVES. 'A horse,' he sighs, 'is just about the most beautiful work of God that breathes.'"

— Cleveland Amory, **The Celebrity Register**, 1963

"From the day STEVE REEVES won the 'Mr. America' trophy, until this day, he has remained... and probably will for all time, the most admired, most looked-up to, and most idolized bodybuilder of all."

— **Muscle Builder**, May 1963

"Vaughn Meader's best selling LP, 'First Family,' has a segment on STEVE REEVES. It seems Jackie, in talking to the president, learns he'd like to see a good Italian movie. Steve Reeves as 'Hercules,' to be exact. Steve has evidently even made a hit with the Kennedy clan!"

— **Muscle Builder**, May 1963

" 'Hercules' was televised for a full week recently on Channel 7. Steve is now living in Switzerland with a cool million salted away in Swiss banks, and of course, all the muscles anyone ever wanted."

— **Muscle Builder**, May 1963

"You admire him as one of the most extravagantly handsome men who ever lived ... the epitome of all high 'Mr. America' standards. To women who have seen him only in photographs or on the screen, he is an implosion of sex; to small fry formerly accustomed to the usual weekly Western he is a living legend, a shining, contemporary knight who embodies the heroism of Hercules, the gallantry of Galahad, and the derring-do of d'Artagnan."

— **Young Physique**, November 1963

"REEVES! REEVES! REEVES! I liked the picture of Steve Reeves you printed. But I hate your column because you showed two pictures of Glenn Bishop and only one of Steve. How can you do this to Steve? How dare you do this to his loyal fans?"

— **Young Physique**, November 1963

" 'Hercules' takes a bride! So popular and well known is STEVE REEVES that his recent marriage to countess Aline Czartawicz in Lucerne, Switzerland was given top priority by the news services. The happy couple's photo appeared in newspapers throughout the world and the event rated television announcements."

— Muscle Builder, March 1964

"STEVE REEVES name is inscribed on the hearts of all who admire a handsome, symmetrical physique. Although Steve is not the most muscular bodybuilder, his memory will be forever in the minds and hearts of all for this reason - Steve was the handsomest of them all. Others have played 'Hercules,' yet none has symbolized the great Hercules as has Steve. Others might be more massive, muscular, or stronger, but they represent crude strongman... the coarse individual... the type of man that the public doesn't especially care for. When other Hercules appear on the screen, we can hardly wait for them to be destroyed — eaten by the lions — so we can get the heck out of the theater. We doubt if anyone will ever come along who embodies the All-American ideal more than Steve Reeves does so completely. Steve has captivated us all! Steve, if you will make a comeback in physical-culture shows, the world of bodybuilding will be greatly rewarded. We will welcome you back, Steve. We miss the greatness of you!"

— **Muscle Builder**, January 1965

"The legendary STEVE REEVES is considered to have the greatest calves of all time, measuring 18-1/2 inches cold with flawless shape."

— **Mr. America**, March 1965

"Men, how would you like to date every beautiful eyeful you set eyes on? You would! Well, all you need is a physique bulging with muscles and, oh yes, a name. Something like STEVE REEVES! Because that's the seven-year record of the husky guy who catapulted to fame as Mr. Hercules himself. Steve has been seen with just about every beautiful face and figure in Europe, and romantically linked with most of them, ever since he migrated to Italy. He has been having the time of his life."

— **Richard Prager**, Midnight, April 5, 1965

"Recently seen in the hills of Scotland was STEVE REEVES. He attended a beef auction to bid for new stock for his ranch."

— **Muscle Builder**, October 1965

"STEVE REEVES was tapped for immortality by an Italian movie director - who prevailed upon him to enact 'Hercules' ... Until this steel door was opened, the muscle boys had nothing to shoot at except a national title and regional homage. Their playing fields were beaches and gymnasiums. The success of Steve Reeves changed all that....Women, as well as men, wanted to see what a real, solid body looked like. Sparked by the dedication of Reeves, some 5,000,000 American men are reputedly enrolled in thousands of gymnasiums, health clubs, reducing salons, and spas. They, too, would like to be as brawny as he is."

— Gerald McCue, **Bachelor**, April 1966

"STEVE 'HERCULES' REEVES visited the all-Morgan show sponsored by the Morgan Horse Club of Southern California held at the Carnation Ring, Pomona, California. He is soon to leave for Spain to film his first Western."

— **Muscle Builder**, September 1966

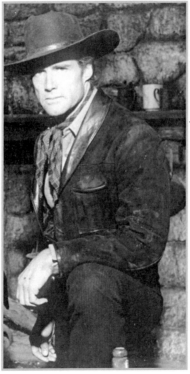

"How famous can you get! STEVE REEVES by marriage is tenth cousin to Princess Radziwill. Princess Radziwill is the sister of Jackie Kennedy. Somehow that makes Steve some sort of relation to our former president."

— **Muscular Development**, April 1967

"Everyone wants to know about STEVE REEVES....His magic has cast a 20-year spell! No male has captured the imagination quite so much as Steve, even amongst the younger physical-culture enthusiasts who never saw him in all his glory....There is a special place for Steve Reeves in the archives of physical-culture. Perhaps it was because he was before his time, for people can look at pictures of him taken 20 years ago, and they have not aged; they could have been taken last week....After Steve's 'Mr. America' victory, he was talked about all over the world. I was in Cyprus in the Army at the time I first saw pictures of Reeves, and I can well remember the sensation they caused."

— Oscar Heidenstam, **Health & Strength**, March 8, 1967

"We had over 1,000 spectators in the grandstand on Saturday night, and among the celebrities in the audience were film stars STEVE REEVES, who attended the whole show, and Kim Novak, who came down from *her Big Sur home."*

— **Morgan Horse**, September 1969

"Congratulations to Mr. and Mrs. STEVE REEVES on the purchase of the lovely weanling filly, Waer's Donlana, who won her first blue ribbon at the Golden West National Morgan Show."

— **Morgan Horse**, September 1969

"Mickey Hagarty recently met STEVE REEVES and reported Steve looking great, though body weight was down."

— Muscle Builder, July 1969

"It is amazing, but twenty years after he won the 'Mr. Universe,' we still receive letters requesting STEVE REEVES' present measurements, training methods, photos, etc....The Reeves magic lives on!"

— Muscle Builder, January 1970

"Next month, a cover shot of the million dollar physique— STEVE REEVES — in a fine pose we believe all fans will like."

— **Muscular Development**, October 1970

"It's for sure that he is the idol of millions. Will it be possible for us to have the chance and happiness of seeing STEVE REEVES, who gives the impression of ancient Greek gods with his magnificent aesthetics, in a contest as guest star?"

— **I.F.B.B. Bulletin**, September 1971

"The incredible STEVE REEVES does it again! A runaway first-place in the bodybuilders popularity poll. We congratulate you, Steve Reeves, wherever you are. There's a beautiful trophy waiting for you at this office."

— **Muscle Builder**, July 1971

"STEVE REEVES, who once flexed his mighty muscles in a series of costume Italian films, looms as a strong possibility to return to the screen as the title hero of the 'Doc Savage' tales George Pal is planning to produce."

— Bob Porter, **Dallas Morning News**, February 19, 1973

"STEVE REEVES was recently the Grand Marshall in the Vista Christmas Parade....Reeves hasn't made a movie in three years and says he won't until the current emphasis on sex and nudity ends."

— **Iron Man**, July 1973

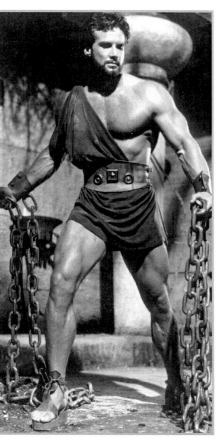

"What brings Levine to Dallas is the reissue of the two films of STEVE REEVES which started the filmmaker's empire, 'Hercules' and 'Hercules Unchained.'....Now it seems box-office lightning will strike twice. The films have already been reissued in San Antonio to strong grosses....'A new generation of moviegoers wants to be exposed to Hercules,' says Levine. 'We proved that in San Antonio. There's a special kind of audience for this kind of picture. The public is always the deciding factor, not the critics.'"

— **Dallas Morning News**, July 27, 1973

"'Hercules' and 'Hercules Unchained,' which are scheduled to go back into a national re-release, start this week in Dallas as the first important opening....'I was sure 'Hercules' was going to be a hit that first time,' said Levine. 'Things were different then and you had some way of knowing the market. I was sure it was going to be very successful. If it hadn't been, it would have been the end of me in this business. I borrowed a lot of money for that picture. You know, 'Hercules' was not made on the grand scale of a 'Ben-Hur,' but if it had been I think it would have been the biggest film of all time. There is something about 'Hercules.' There are people who know of 'Hercules' who never heard

of 'Ben-Hur'...Levine is hoping to get STEVE REEVES, who starred in both pictures, to head the publicity tour, but Reeves, who has become a cult-figure in muscle building circles because of his fine muscle proportions rather than muscle bulk, still hasn't made up his mind."

— Don Safran, Dallas Times Herald, July 29, 1973

"His bank account bulges as much as his muscles, and so at 47, STEVE REEVES, filmland's 'Hercules,' is still on top of it. After living in Switzerland, tall, tan, trim, Reeves moved to a 14-acre spread last year and settled down with his petite, blonde wife, Aline. There, in a modern sprawling, comfortable house surrounded by fruit orchards, he does only what he wants to, as befits a former 'Hercules.' After starring in 16 movies between 1957 and 1968 without a shirt on his back, he can now afford to keep it covered quite well because he invested his money wisely....For a man who once withstood the outrageous slings and arrows of numerous Italian costume epics, the world is a peaceful place....He doesn't particularly enjoy contact with his fans anymore. 'I've been in the public eye for the last 30 years,' he explained. 'The more you're in the public eye, the more you value your privacy.' Still, fans of his movies and bodybuilders continue to call, write and even stop by unannounced. He did welcome a rabbi from Dallas, Texas who wanted advice on bodybuilding. 'He was kosher and brought along bagels, lox, and cream cheese, so we had a good time eating and discussing philosophy.' "

— Martin Gerchen, **Copley News Service**, August 28, 1973

"STEVE REEVES, the muscular former 'Mr. Universe' who became an overnight sensation in 'Hercules' roles during the 1950s, starred in 16 movies and made a fortune. Today he raises horses on his own hilltop ranch. 'I'm happier here on the ranch riding and breeding horses than I ever was on a movie set,' said Reeves....'This is what I've always dreamed of having. I never planned to stay in movies all my life. They were always a means to an end for me....I enjoyed making films but no one can go on forever...It was inevitable that a new trend in public tastes would come along eventually.' "

— Jolyon Wilde, **National Enquirer**, November 25, 1973

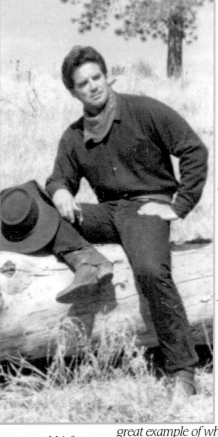

"As a result of wise stock market investments throughout his film career, two years ago STEVE REEVES fulfilled a lifelong ambition by retiring at age 45. A unique physical specimen by any standards, the screen giant remains in top shape by jogging and swimming ....'Most men retire at 65, but I wanted to retire at 45, giving me 20 extra years,' says Reeves. 'Look at Tyrone Power and Errol Flynn — they never had those extra years.' "

— Marty Gunther, **Tattler**, December 16, 1973

"New York City welcomed STEVE REEVES with thunderous applause, from the moment his plane touched down right until the time he stepped off the WBBG dais on the night of the show.... I was glad to wait until the big American Airliner touched down from San Diego, California and see for the first time this truly great example of what we all want to achieve in our lifetime....This quiet man of the outdoors sat proudly, and was obviously very knowledgeable in his first TV appearance on the A.M. New York Show as he was interviewed by comic Soupy Sales and 'Mr. Warmth' of the sports world, Howard Cosell. The show was on Channel 7 on Friday September 7, and was seen by millions. We shared an hour with Joe Franklin on his Memory Lane WOR-TV show on Channel 9 next, and Steve was accorded an honor that Joe Franklin reserved for 'one of the greatest movie box-office attractions of all-time.' It was repeated five times due to viewer demand!....Friday afternoon Dan Lurie arranged a meeting with the office of the Commissioner of Public Events where Deputy Commissioner Milito welcomed Steve Reeves and his wife to our city and told them that the award of the Key to the City was the first time such an honor had been given 'to a great physical culturist' and that New York was indeed proud to have Reeves in our midst 'in this time of great unrest, when our youth sorely needs guidance and inspiration.'...At Randalls Island, Commissioner Davidson gave Steve the Key to the City and a copy of the proclamation declaring Saturday September 8, 1973 as Physical Culture Day in honor of Steve Reeves....Steve and Mrs. Reeves received a standing ovation when he was introduced by his good friend Tony Aguilar, the star of the Mexican Horse Show at Madison Square Garden on Saturday afternoon....We headed for the big event of Steve's trip the WBBG 1973 'Mr. America/Mr. World Show at Hunter College, where the largest audience ever to be crowded into that auditorium welcomed the 'Guru of Physical Culture' for so many years. The contests proceeded well to an appreciative, overcrowded, standing room only audience, but the tension mounted when two 'Hercules' film clips were shown. Our guest of honor stepped out on the stage and at that moment no one in the crowded auditorium could hold back his enthusiasm. Dan Lurie's presentation of the WBBG Honor Award was made, and then Steve's words of gratitude echoed his feelings. 'If I have been a source of inspiration for many of you in these past years, then I am happy to have been, and deeply grateful that you have seen fit to honor me.' Steve Reeves had come all the way back in one brief appearance that very moment. He is a man deserving of every accolade we have all seen fit to bestow upon him.

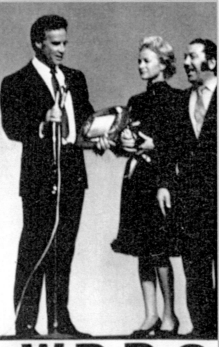

— Nat Haber, **Muscle Training Illustrated**, December 1973

"STEVE REEVES had just arrived at New York's Kennedy Airport....Steve Reeves will be here any minute,' Nat Haver tells the crowd. 'He looks terrific. A little gray, distinguished, like Billy Graham....We should all look like that at 47!.... Steve Reeves entered the press room ... Everyone stood in applause, flashbulbs popping. Reassuringly, Reeves is not four-feet eleven, his stomach is not hanging over his belt. He is six-foot-one and handsome, though certainly bearing no resemblance to Billy Graham. The green suit fits a little tight but presumably that happens when you have one of those chests, and anyway everything crescendos and tapers off at the right points. He looks like the perfect businessman. He and his wife, an attractive, blonde woman, took seats ....'Did you use a special diet when you were training, Steve?' [He answered] 'When I had a 'Volkswagon body I put Volkswagon fuel into it; when I had a Cadillac body I put Cadillac fuel into it.'...'What do you attribute your success to?' 'I was able to concentrate. When I started I exhausted myself one day, then rested two. I got an inch bigger every day.' Applause. 'Did you have any heroes, Steve?' 'No one person. I chose parts of different people, the thighs of one male, the arms of another. 'Moderator: 'What we have here then is a collage of all the best-built people in the world!' "

— Robert Strozier, **Atlantic Monthly**, March 1974

"I have known Steve since he was seventeen. He has a tremendous knowledge of kinesiology, nutrition and special exercises. He is a man of the highest integrity and forthrightness and practices what he preaches."

— Jack LaLanne, **PowerWalking**, 1982

"Physically he is a genetic phenomenon, standing over six feet, with the world's most classic physique and a face as handsome as *any movie star. Steve Reeves is truly one of a kind."*

— Armand Tanny, **Muscle & Fitness**, May 1983

"Handsome and with a physique that set new standards for bodybuilding, the truly unique Steve Reeves fueled athletic fantasies for thousands of youngsters through his roles in "Hercules," "The Last Days Of Pompeii" and other films. M&F proudly profiles this still-active fitness leader now enjoying a productive private life."

— **Muscle & Fitness**, May 1983

"I became aware of Steve Reeves about 1946. In 1947, when he won the Mr. America in Chicago, he was the best-looking man — from every perspective: facially, physically, everything — who I think probably ever lived up to that time. In the first place he's about 6-foot-1-inch, extremely broad shouldered. And the guy was just incredibly handsome. Reeves is the first guy that epitomized the term "beautiful body." When I was out at Muscle Beach in California in 1957, he'd be down at the beach and the little groupies that came down to the beach on weekends would just line up to look at Steve Reeves.

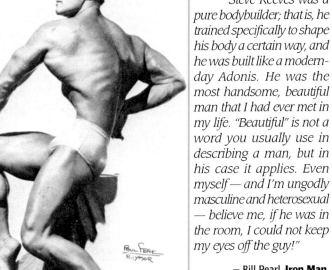

I'll tell you another thing about him. He trained his physique so it wound up producing that kind of body. He did exercises like hack squats, and he preferred exercises like dumbbell inclines over bench presses. He was extremely good at using angles. I remember he used to do this big curl movement, seated dumbbell curls, on about a 45-degree angle so that it worked all the way up into the high insertion up under the anterior deltoid when you contracted at the top. He knew his body exquisitely, and he got exactly the kind of results that kind of training was designed to produce."

— George Turner, **Iron Man**, May 1995

"Steve Reeves' physique is perfect. Fantastic physique. Not that huge body, but it was so perfect, so lean, that it became something incredible. Because every muscle, every tendon was perfect — from his calves to his head. Very good proportions. Tremendous symmetry. And such a tremendous looking man. Well, this man has been good looking, I think, since the day he came out of his mom. He'd go crazy on the stage, and the women go crazy.... I had the pleasure and opportunity to travel with Steve Reeves when I was conducting seminars all over Europe and he was invited as a guest. I found out that not only his physique is wonderful, he is a wonderful man. [I've got a] lot of experience in this game of bodybuilding, and I respect the man even more now that we had an opportunity to share time together."

— Sergio Oliva, **Iron Man**, May 1995

"Steve Reeves was a pure bodybuilder; that is, he trained specifically to shape his body a certain way, and he was built like a modern-day Adonis. He was the most handsome, beautiful man that I had ever met in my life. "Beautiful" is not a word you usually use in describing a man, but in his case it applies. Even myself — and I'm ungodly masculine and heterosexual — believe me, if he was in the room, I could not keep my eyes off the guy!"

— Bill Pearl, **Iron Man**, May 1995

(The following excerpts are from the book, "Steve Reeves One of a Kind," by Milton T. Moore, Jr. (c) 1983)

"I first saw Steve in 1946. A friend and I were attending a contest in Berkeley. The theatre was jammed, standing room only. Then just before curtain time, eveyone's heads started turning and people began standing. And down the aisle walked this big, young good-looking soldier, in Army woolen trousers and matching shirt...there's nothing uglier...paratrooper boots, black tie...no cap...and he looked like something

form outer space. All heads were looking at Steve; the auditorium was rumbling. Everyone was asking: 'Who is that?' And we finally found out it was Steve Reeves. He was absolutely fantastic, and anyone sitting there—and it was my opinion too—had to be thinking that this guy's got to be a winner; he's going to be a superstar in whatever he does....and he looked all of 18 or 19 years old. And Steve wasn't involved in the show in any way. He was on leave from the Army; had bought a ticket like the rest of us; and was just looking for a seat....and the audience went wild. Steve hadn't even started [competing] yet....He just had that big, good looking, raw-bone, fantastic, natural physique, although he had been working out—no doubt."

—Joe Corsi, 1946

"I don't think there is one chance in 50 trillion that the particular mix of hereditary genes that produced the product we see in Steve Reeves will ever occur in combination again. Steve was a very unusual bodybuilder. He had the overall beauty that no other bodybuilder has ever been able to achieve. I have had the occasion to work with, photographically, most of the top bodybuilders in the world. But when the good Lord made Steve Reeves, he threw the mold away. There has never been another man, as we go back through all written word and graphic representation, who...ever came out like Steve did. He is from another galaxie.

"I'll never forget one evening when Steve accompanied Jack LaLanne and I to a restaurant. When Steve entered the room, everyone stopped eating. You could hear the knives and forks drop. Some people froze with their mouths open. They looked at him in amazement, as if he were a man from another world. Of course, 99-percent of them had never heard of Steve Reeves and thought he was a movie star. And this was the case wherever Steve set foot: there was admiration from the men, the women and even the little children.

"Let's face it: there is only one Steve Reeves. He's an original. I consider it my privilege to have been alive in that period of time when I had the association with Steve. I know as the years roll by, and we are all gone, Steve will live on in history as the greatest of all time in the field of physical culture, in addition to being one of the finest human beings ever created."

—Russ Warner

Steve participated in the 1948 Mr. Universe Contest staged in London on August 23. Steve Reeves' fame proceeded him as thousands of physical culture enthusiasts crowded into London to watch him compete for the first time in Europe....British movie star, Patricia Plunket, posed with Steve after the contest, in which Steve placed second to John Grimek. But Steve was first in the hearts and minds of many, including King Frederick IX of Denmark, who wanted Steve to be his personal physical instructor. King Frederick, whose favorite pastime was guest-conducting symphony orchestras, realized that Steve Reeves, like a Stradivarius, could never be replaced.

—Milton Moore, 1948

"Steve was very serious in his work; showed tremendous discipline and engaged himself in a hard way. He moved into the character he played and lived there. Although "Hercules" was his first starring role, Steve was sure of himself. And an actor is acting well only when he feels sure of himself.

"Steve Reeves was the most naturally glamorous start of any period in the cinema. As a painter and sculptor, my qualifications governing the selection of the man to portray "Hercules" were taken from Michelangelo, in my subconscious. Consequently, I chose Steve because he had an alarmingly handsome face that blended perfectly with history's most spectacular physique. Through the expression of his face he could communicate to audiences that his mind was deep in thought and far way from the events that were occurring around him. He seemed at times to be contemplating things beyond the comprehension of ordinary individuals, as a god, a god that had descended from something far above the cosmos known to the everyday filmgoer.

"The background for my "Hercules" films were the ancient Greek poems, "Le Argonauti" by Rodio, and "I Sette Atebe," by Eschilo. Without the presence of Steve Reeves, the translation of these poems into film, as the poems themselves, would have been vital and relevant only to a meager, scholarly audience. However, Steve Reeves gave the Greek poems the extra dimension they needed to animate and popularize them for everyone worldwide. Through Steve millions of people received this culture without even realizing it.

"Steve, now in his fifties, has a face that projects even more force, fixed intelligence and honest determination than twenty years ago. The passage of time has etched in an interesting, commanding rugged look. His is a face to build another epic around."

—Pietro Francisci, 1970s

"As far as international publicity and everything involved in the image of bodybuilders, no one else has ever topped Steve Reeves. Of course, we still have another twenty-one years before this century is completed, but I double that Reeves will ever be topped. You might call him the MAN OF THE TWENTIETH CENTURY."

—Tony Lanza, 1979

Dr. Avard Fairbanks, a Guggenheim Fellow and one of the world's leading art figures, is renown as the world's greatest sculptor of Lincoln, and is the executor of over 90 major works on various subjects, including the Great Chicago Lincoln; the Fighting Siox Monument; the Poney Express Monument; the Pioneer Family Group Monument; and the statue of Lycurgus, still displayed in Sparta, Greece.

Dr. Fairbanks comments on Steve Reeves: "The design of the human system is to bring oneself in line with the same harmonies that regulate the universe. It is these underlying forms and harmonies that elevate man's life and man's thinking. Steve Reeves is the epitome of a man bringing his physique into harmony with the universe he is a part of. He's the grandest example I have ever seen of Michelangelo's dream come true. It is unfortunate Steve Reeves was not living during the Renaissance period, for the Masters would have worn their hands to the bone making statues from him."

—Avard Fairbanks, Sculptor

Perhaps my most poignant memory of Steve was when he and I rode a bus up to a very popular summer spot on the Russian River, called "Rio Nido." We rented a room at a motor court and spent the day canoeing, swimming and sunbathing...That evening we attended the dance. We entered the large hall, which was in the middle of a large grove of redwoods, walked over to the rows of benches and sat down, just the two of us, quietly waiting for the music to start. When the music began, suddenly girls appeared from everywhere and converged on Steve, sitting on either side of him, and one even sat on his lap. all of them looking at him amiringly. We didn't know any of them....Without speaking a word, he jumped up and left the building. All that attention was just too much. He still didn't consider himself anything special...or unique. I returned to...our room a couple of hours later, Steve was sleeping peacefully. And I remember how he looked in sleep. Here was a guy who looked better sleeping...than do all of the millions of would-be bodybuilding idols when they are up on stage—trained, tanned, oiled and tensed. And I remember thinking to myself: 'What a waistline on that guy, what fantastic bone-structure, what symmetry!' Unstaged and unrehearsed and not conscious of being observed, here was a great Bengal tiger in repose.

I never mentioned it to Steve, but even then I knew that Steve Reeves was destined to attain heights where no man has stood before or since."

—Clem Poechmann—Boyhood friend from the 1940s

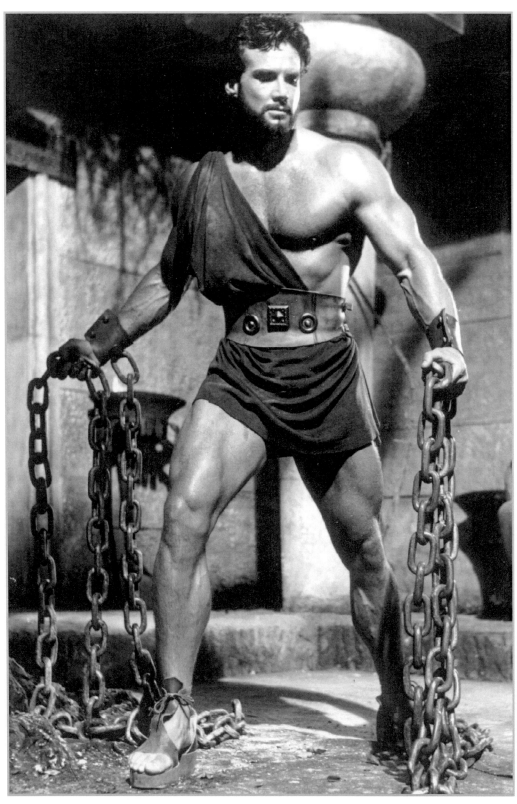

"The star of 'Hercules Unchained' is a young man of muscle named Steve Reeves, who is something of a phenomenon...an amazing set of muscles..." St. Louis Post-Dispatch.

Appendix 7

In their own words –– Impressions of Steve Reeves from Mentors and Friends

The Making of a Champion
by Alyce Stagg Yarick, 1947

Those of you who were fortunate in being in Chicago on the 29th of June 1947, saw Steve Reeves presented with the highest honor bestowed on any bodybuilder — Mr. America. It is the title for America's most perfectly developed physique which was achieved only through exercise and healthy living. What is more important than one's health?

Some of you may have seen his photos in your local newspaper or in a newsreel. But for those of you who missed out, let me tell you, Steve is something to see! A blue eyed lad, he stands 6-feet-1-inch tall and weighs 213 pounds. He is handsome — and I do mean handsome! When he smiles you can feel his warm personality and his boyish charm.

Steve was unknown until he won a contest in Portland in December 1946 — and even then we heard little about him! Steve had high hopes and was working for a much bigger goal so he gave very little information about himself. A shy lad, he felt that a media build up now could lead to a letdown later so, he didn't want any stories written about him.

Steve started training at the age of 16. He was a tall well-built boy with good bone structure. One day he visited a friend named Joe Gambina. Joe and a few other friends were having a arm-wrestling contest, and Steve decided to try his strength. He challenged Joe but Joe beat him. This puzzled Steve. How could a light boy, a much smaller boy like Joe, be able to take him down? He asked Joe what made him so strong. Joe showed Steve the weights he had in his garage. Steve trained a short time with Joe, for which Joe charge him 50 cents a workout. Finally on his own, with determination to go after the top award, he trained and trained hard.

Steve then started to collect strength and health magazines to learn all he could about bodybuilding. Weight training to Steve was like baseball, football or basketball to other enthusiastic athletes. Each youngster is eager to reach the highest goal in their chosen field — baseball, the big leagues and football, collegiate or professional ball. Steve's goal was to be Mr. America.

Steve needed the help of a knowledgable bodybuilder who could guide him in the right direction. He chose Ed Yarick and trained under Ed's supervision for two years before being drafted. Steve was inducted into the Army on September 16, 1944 and had six weeks of basic training before being sent to the Philippines, where he joined the 25th Infantry Division.... He was discharged two years and two months from the time he was inducted.... As soon as he arrived home, he returned to Yarick's and again trained with Ed. He regularly trained under Ed's instruction until the Mr. America contest in Chicago. Steve trained three days a week without fail. He hit the workouts hard and never missed one.

Steve actually did miss a workout one Saturday in December of 1946....On the following Tuesday, Steve's next workout day, Steve walked into Yarick's gym holding a trophy. The trophy read, "Steve Reeves - Mr. Pacific Coast of 1946, Portland Oregon."... He then planned to be a participant in the Mr. Western America contest held in Los Angeles. Steve did not enter the Mr. California contest as he had just won the larger contest. Eric Pederson won the Mr. California contest and later placed second to Steve in both the Mr. Western America and the Mr. America.

After winning the Mr. Western America contest in 1947 (where he received 72 points out of a possible 75), Steve had only one goal yet to achieve — the Mr. America title. With this goal held consistently in mind, Steve's determination became stronger than ever. Ed was an excellent workout coach who combined his knowledge of physiology with an innate understanding of psychology to guide and encourage each person to reach their potential.

Steve's mother was supportive and helped him in every way she could as Steve's enthusiasm and determination grew. Like any mother, she wanted what was best for her son. She cooked his meals as he wanted. Alhough he was not fussy, he preferred plenty of salads, meat, vegetables, milk and eggs. He always drank at least one quart of milk a day. Steve did not eat white bread, white flour products, candy or white sugar. He liked lots of fresh fruits and used honey for his sweets.

He retired early every night assuring he would get enough sleep. Steve wasn't just exercising, he was exercising strenuously, and needed the proper rest to rebuild tissues. Besides, he was always very active: horseback riding, cycling, hiking, ice skating and doing ranch-chores for his uncle in Montana (when he wasn't training for a contest). Steve also benefitted from this regime in other ways: he never had to see a doctor — he was always in perfect health, and at 21 years old, he never had a cavity.

Steve's mother felt her efforts were rewarded — especially by the titles Steve won. She shared her son's happiness and was also happy for the kindness people showed him. Mothers like Steve's help make champions.

To our Mr. America, weight training is like a science and he enjoys the exercising. He utilizes a well-balanced routine using strict form — no bouncing, swinging or cheating of any kind. As a body builder, Steve did not participate in Olympic or heavy weightlifting. Bodybuilders train differently than weightlifters — although Steve built up to half squats with 400 pounds, using 75 pound dumbbells in each hand on the incline curls, 110 pound dumbbells on the incline presses, 20 repetitions on the calf raises with 450 pounds.

Steve has narrow hips, broad shoulders, a small waist and beautifully proportioned legs. He is a handsome young man who reminds us of Lil' Abner. With his terrific personality and perfect health, who could be more suitable to hold the title of Mr. America!

— • —

Steve's measurements when he joined Ed's gym at age 16 and at age 21 (one month before he won the Mr. America title):

	At 16 Years	At 21 Years
Weight	163 pounds	213 pounds
Height	6-foot	6-foot-1-inch
Neck	13-1/2"	17-3/4"
Chest Normal	37"	49-1/2"
Chest Expanded	39-1/2"	51"
Waist	30"	29"
Thighs	22-1/2"	25-1/2"
Calf	16"	18"
Biceps	13-1/2"	18"

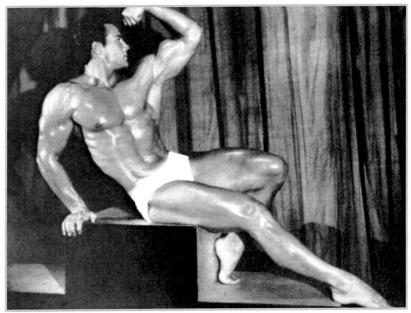
1948 Mr. World competitionn in Cannes, France.

The Steve Reeves I Know and Remember
By Ed Yarick

Reeves is universally known as the "Hercules" of the movies. He won Mr. America, Mr. World and Mr. Universe titles, yet few know much about him as a person. Just who is he? How did he get started in bodybuilding? How did he train?

My association with Steve goes back over 30 years. In the 40s, my Oakland, California gym was located near three high schools — Oakland, Fremont and Castlemont. Reeves attended Castlemont (one of the few schools of that era that had a set of weights). He began working out at school and at home but spent much of his free time touring local bodybuilding gyms and trying to obtain all possible information about bodybuilding. During this period, he stopped at my gym and decided to train under my supervision, gaining 30 pounds of solid muscle in four months.

For two years, Steve worked out with my instructions and encouragement. His progress continued to be outstanding. By the time he was eighteen, Reeves weighed a solid 203 pounds. The opinion of many experts was if he entered the Mr. America that year, he could win the title. His physique was already showing signs of the fine shape and muscularity that would eventually make him the most famous bodybuilder of our time.

Steve graduated from Castlemont in 1944, at the height of World War II, and was inducted into the Army. At that time, soldiers were quickly shipped overseas, and Reeves was no exception. After six short weeks of basic training, he was shipped out to fight in the Philippines where he earned the Combat Infantryman's Badge and several other medals. During that time, however, he contracted a severe case of malaria, requiring a long period of hospitalization and resulting in a weight loss of more than 20 pounds. After several recurrences, Steve was finally transferred from combat duty to the quartermaster corps. He eventually ended up in Japan with General McArthur's occupation troops.

Steve was still recuperating from his malaria attacks in 1946 and was physically well below par. He had not had a bodybuilding workout in more than a year, and with no available equipment, it didn't look as if he would be able to train again. But in typical Reeves' *find-a-way-or-make-one* fashion, he located an interpreter to take with him to a local foundry. With the aid of sketches and much hand-waving, Steve was able to have a 250-pound barbell set made up. With this equipment, he began training again. It wasn't long before he had a regular gym set up and a number of other soldiers exercising with him.

We kept in touch by mail, and in the fall of 1946, he was discharged and return home. Without delay he was back training in my gym, but this time he was no longer a pupil. Instead we were workout partners, training diligently three times a week on a routine that included several exercises that Steve had invented. These sessions continued as regularly as clock work and were something we both look forward to. I was improving and I could see Steve rapidly growing in size and shape. He never missed workouts, so I was surprised when Steve didn't show for one of his regular Saturday sessions. I was extremely puzzled because he was in such top condition that he simply could not have been ill.

I found out the reason when he showed up for his Tuesday workout and gave me a huge trophy inscribed, "Mr. Pacific Coast of 1946" to display in the gym window. Without telling anyone, Steve and his new workout partner, Bob Weidlich, took a train to Portland, Oregon, and entered the contest. That's how Steve is. He never sought publicity and didn't even desire any advanced buildup prior to his Mr. America victory.

Early in January of 1947, a Mr. California contest was held. Steve didn't enter, having won the larger Mr. Pacific Coast title a month earlier. Instead he entered and won the Mr. Western America. He took home trophies at that event for Best Arms, Best Legs and Best Chest. Then after three months of hard training, Steve won the big one — the Mr. America title in Chicago.

Many bodybuilding fans have asked me about Steve Reeves early years. He was born in Montana on January 21, 1926, and is of Welsh, Irish, English and German descent. His father died when Steve was a year and a half old. Reeves attended boarding schools and spent summers on his uncle's ranch in Montana. Steve learned to ride when he was 3 years old and is an excellent horseman. When he was 10, Steve and his mother moved to Oakland.

To do his share in helping out financially, Steve had a newspaper route. He was proud of being the only one among the carriers who could pedal his bike up the steep East Oakland hills with a full load of papers. The rest were obliged to walk and push their loaded bikes up the hill, but Steve always made it a point to pedal up. He gives much credit to his strenuous bike exercise for his early leg development. His calves are truly exceptional in size and contour. I would say that even as a boy a Steve was physique conscious because he would pedal that bike in a manner designed to provide his legs with the greatest amount of stimulation.

One of Steve's greatest supporters was his mother, Goldie. She encouraged his athletic endeavors, and always made sure that he had nutritious, well-balanced meals. Steve is especially fond of steak, salad, vegetables, fresh fruits and nuts. He consumed more than a quart of milk a day when I knew him. He never smoked, drank alcoholic beverages or ate any products containing devitalized white flour or refined white sugar. He substituted honey for sugar. As a result of his healthy diet, Reeves teeth are a dental advertisement, totally free from cavities.

Our training program was a very strenuous one. We adhered to a three-day-per-week schedule and had no favorite exercises. Instead, we employed a broad variety of exercises in an effort to arrive at a well-balanced physique. Steve did not endeavor to specialize in competitive lifts, but the very heavy poundages and high repetitions that he employed in bodybuilding exercises provided plenty of evidence that he was exceptionally powerful.

Steve used a very strict form in all of our exercise movements. We did each exercise from complete extension to complete contraction, no swinging, no bouncing, no cheating of any kind. It did not matter to us if we only did seven or eight reps with our heaviest weights as long as each rep was done in perfect style.

I will briefly describe one of the routines Steve and I would use. We started with exercises for the deltoids (shoulders) to attain a wide look in that area and followed these with moments for the pectorals (chest). Then we moved to the latissimus dorsi (upper back) which gives a "V" shaped, tapered appearance to the torso, the biceps and triceps (upper arms), the thighs and calves (legs), the lower back and the neck. As mentioned before, we always did a variety of exercises to promote all around development.

Outside the gym, Steve and I shared many good times together. During the warm summer months, many Bay area bodybuilders would gather at Sunny Cove Beach in Alameda, just a short distance from Oakland. We would bask in the sun and swim either in the surf or an adjacent pool. Jack LaLanne and I hand-balanced a lot, while my wife Alyce and many of the local barbell enthusiasts talked and exchanged views on bodybuilding. Steve was always one of the of most ardent in all of these discussions.

In the winter months, we had an occasional "Sunday meeting" at the of local ice skating rink. Wearing a ski sweater over his wide-shouldered and narrow-hipped "V" shape along with his natural good looks, Steve was always the main attraction of our group. The girls did double-takes as they passed by him, and after a while, they seemed to pass by him quite frequently. He was truly an all-American boy.

Reeves is always inclined to be a bit modest. Steve is intelligent and has both high ideals and a conscientious nature. He was also very unselfish, especially in the way he encourage youngsters in bodybuilding. I knew there would be nothing to stop Steve from going on to bigger and better things, and of course no one is more deserving of success then he.

I was confident he would go on to accomplish a tremendous amount of good on behalf of the of physical culture movement. I knew that one day Steve would leave Oakland — the Southern California beaches had more to offer him. He no longer needed instruction. But he did need the opportunities in television and film offered in Los Angeles. I wished him well and he was off to seek his fortune.

Alyce and I stayed in touch with Steve and would see him along with many of his friends when he dropped by his folks' house. He liked to go into the kitchen and help with the of broiling of steaks or making a tossed salad, as these were his favorite foods. I remember how appreciative he was when we gave him a blender to mix his high-protein health drinks.

Steve went on to win Mr. World and Mr. Universe before devoting himself to acting. He later toured with stage plays like "Kismet," "Wish You Were Here" and "The Vamp" with Carol Channing. His first big movie break came in "Athena" with Jane Powell and Debbie Reynolds. He starred in 16 movies, his most popular being "Hercules." I have always said that Steve's physique was much like a drawing of Lil' Abner, the sort of All-American ideal admired by the general public. We've yet to see another like him, with his handsome face, a keen mind and the most classic physique of all time. He was and is the one and only Steve Reeves!

—— • ——

How Steve Reeves Trained

By John C. Grimek

On Memorial Day May 30, 1950, Steve Reeves arrived in York (Muscletown), Pennsylvania, with his workout partner George Eiferman to train for the upcoming Mr. Universe Contest. We had dinner and then located a place for them to stay. They both were a little tired from the long, across country trip and wanted to start training the following day.

The next morning, Reeves and Eiferman walked into the old barbell building at the York gym, eager for a good workout. It was obvious that Steve had not trained for sometime. Reeves asked whether a specialty T-bar could be made for him so he could utilize his hack squad principle. Jules Bacon, the machine shop manager, not only accomplished this but also fashioned a long cable pulley device for Steve to do seated rowing for his latissimus. Steve took a special liking to our homemade incline bench on which he performed his curls.

The accepted opinion of the fellows in the gym was that he didn't have a chance of winning Mr. Universe. I, too, had my doubts at that time, but we underestimated Reeves' ambition and drive. In a week of training, he began to regain some of his shape. With each workout he took, he put everything into it and continued to do a little more each week. By the end of the second week, Reeves had made remarkable improvement. After working out hard for three weeks, Steve had recovered his large, sinewy arms and a fuller, rounded chest. His back looked wider and more massive. Even his shoulders looked thicker. His abdomen showed more detail and muscularity. Those who saw him train, noticed the dynamic effort he put into each and every workout. He didn't sit around talking and killing time. Instead, he went from one exercise to another. He knew the time was getting short before he would be vying for the Mr. Universe title. He put everything into his training. There was no more whispering in the gym about whether he could win. Everybody agreed it would take a darn good man to beat him now — if he could be beaten!

With each workout, Reeves would increase his training doing more reps, more sets or doing a combination of the two. One of his favorite exercises in York was the curl on the incline bench which he did every workout. After couple weeks, his arms showed the effects of such curling. He also favored the long cable rowing exercise. However, he did this exercise differently from the way most of us perform it. He would bend his body forward and maintain his position while he pulled the bar to his chest by arm and lat power alone, and then he would resist the weight by letting it back slowly. Through his training clothes, we could see his lats and biceps bulge. Another exercise he enjoyed doing was the hack lift. He fixed the platform exactly the way he wanted it, and by using the custom-made long T-bar, he was able to utilize his hack principle and improve the detail of his legs.

During training he had no regard for time, but worked until he had completed his routine — which took anywhere from two to three hours. Of course he came to York to train, so all of his time was devoted to training and resting and this paid off. He would rest only after he finished his training and had his shower. Then he would joke around with the guys.

Now that he was achieving his best possible shape, we spent several evenings developing a suitable posing routine. But time was up, and to our thinking, Steve was ready. He took one final workout and then asked us to appraise his posing. As we watched him shift from one pose to another, it was evident that here was the winner. The improvement he made was amazing. He had worked hard and long those past four weeks and was ready for the big competition.

The following morning, I drove him to the airport in New York and saw him off. A couple of days later, I got word of his victory and was back at the New York airport to greet him and congratulate him as he disembarked. We were as happy over his victory as he was, so we threw a banquet in his honor to celebrate. He was delighted but after a couple of days he bought himself a Ford convertible and began the long drive back California.

Yes, we have watched many a Mr. America and a Mr. Universe train in our old gym, but none whipped themselves into championship shape in less than a month except Reeves.

—— • ——

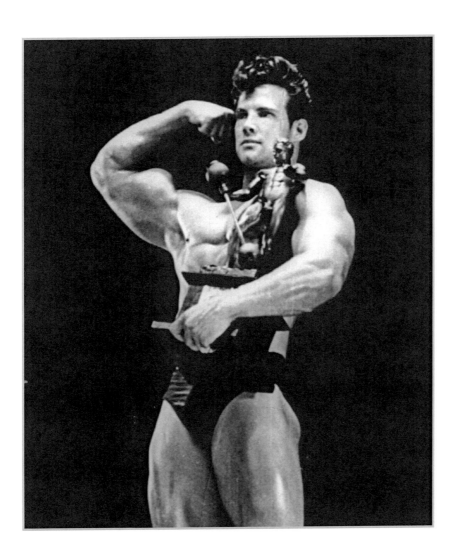

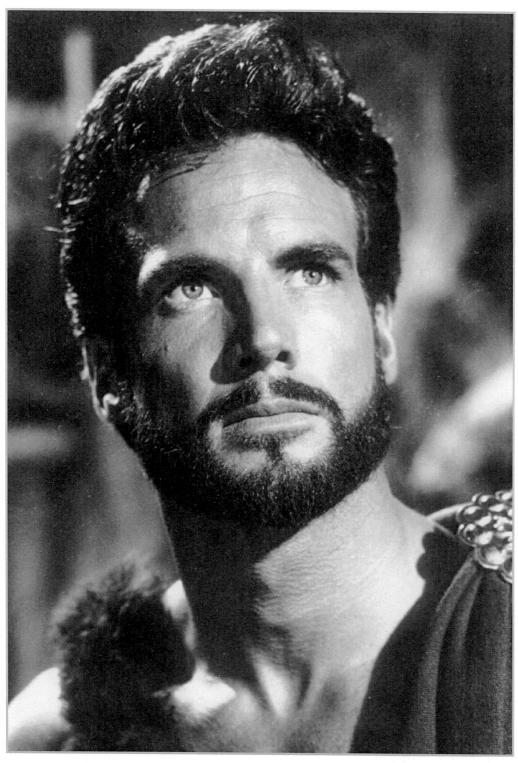

"...my qualifications governing the selection of the man to portray 'Hercules' were taken from Michelangelo in my subconscious; consequently, I chose Steve Reeves because he had an alarmingly handsome face that blended perfectly with history's most spectacular physique."

Director/Producer Pietro Francesci

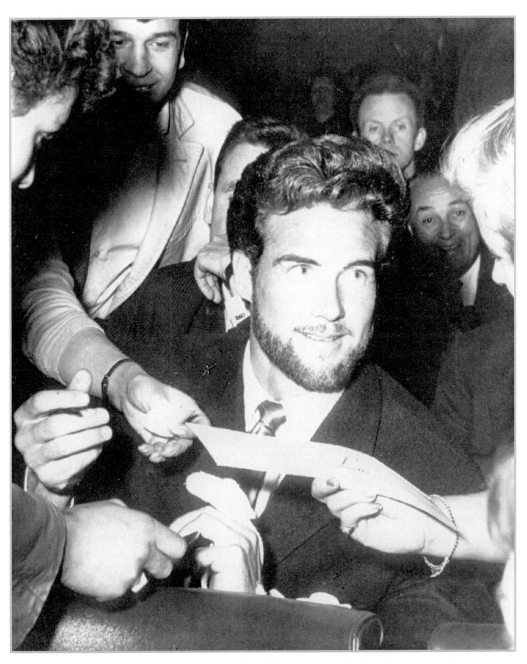
A powerful star worldwide, Steve cheerfully appeases his fans for autographs.

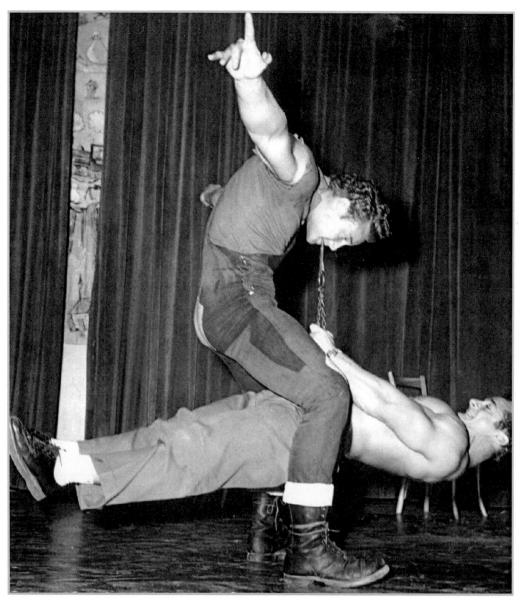

*After performing **Lil' Abner**, Steve performs a unique feat of strength by lifting George Eifferman (weighing over 200 pounds) with his teeth — Santa Monica 1948.*